DEMENTIA AND AGING

DEMENTIA AND AGING
Ethics, Values, and Policy Choices

EDITED BY

Robert H. Binstock, Ph.D.
Stephen G. Post, Ph.D.
Peter J. Whitehouse, M.D., Ph.D.

THE JOHNS HOPKINS UNIVERSITY PRESS
BALTIMORE AND LONDON

The Johns Hopkins University Press
701 West 40th Street
Baltimore, Maryland 21211-2190
The Johns Hopkins Press Ltd., London

Library of Congress Cataloging-in-Publication Data

Dementia and aging : ethics, values, and policy choices / edited by
   Robert H. Binstock, Stephen G. Post, and Peter J. Whitehouse.
      p.   cm.
   Includes bibliographical references and index.
      ISBN 0-8018-4424-X. — ISBN 0-8018-4545-9 (pbk.)
      1. Senile dementia—Treatment—Moral and ethical aspects.
   2. Senile dementia—Treatment—Government policy—United
   States.   3. Senile dementia—Patients—Care—Moral and ethical
   aspects.   4. Senile dementia—Patients—Care—Government
   policy—United States.   I. Binstock, Robert H.   II. Post,
   Stephen Garrard, 1951-.   III. Whitehouse, Peter J.
      [DNLM: 1. Alzheimer's Disease.   2. Dementia, Senile.
   3. Ethics, Medical.   4. Health Policy.   WT 150 D3752]
   RC524.D44 1992
   616.89'83—dc20
   DNLM/DLC
   for Library of Congress   92-6220

CONTENTS

FOREWORD

All human actions have a moral dimension, including actions generated by people with pathological disorders. Certain disorders provoke moral questions, even profound questions about the meaning of life itself. Such is dementia, especially in its advanced stages when it seriously jeopardizes the faculties we ordinarily define as uniquely human: memory, personality, recognition, awareness, the capacity to love, even a sense of hope. The brain, the mind, the spirit, and the will (and we need not make obviously important distinctions here), which constitute the central locus of humanity, are affected. Their loss, next to the total loss of self (i.e., death), is the most frightening specter confronting human beings.

For centuries, it was thought that "senility" or the loss of mental function was the inevitable, natural consequence of aging itself. But since the middle of the twentieth century, it has become more and more apparent that "senility" must give way to more definitive medical diagnoses of a variety of dementias and deliria. These are the vascular form and the parenchymal form of dementia, which predominantly include Alzheimer's disease, of which there are many types. Hidden within the realization that "senility" indicates disease and not inevitability is a message of hope, inasmuch as defining a condition as a disease offers prospects for understanding its genesis, prevention, and treatment. Such has been the case since Hippocrates and others began attributing disease to physical causes rather than divine or demonic ones.

Recently, there have been some groundbreaking advances in dementia research. One of the most stimulating areas of biomedical study concerns the intersection of age and disease, the so-called age-related diseases. Studies of dementia may be facilitated in the future by the production of new research animal models, which might contribute to understanding Alzheimer's disease. Research is benefiting from the new biology, including recombinant DNA, hybridoma and transgenic technologies, and new means of probing the interior of the brain from a distance (computerized axial tomography and magnetic resonance imaging). Perhaps most notable is the prospect of neuroplasticity, the arresting notion that even in old age the brain can heal and repair itself.

Exciting as all this is, however, it is important to realize that, despite progress in our understanding of the central nervous system and its pathologies, including the dementias, we will not have solutions very soon. We must, therefore, confront considerable political, economic, moral, ethical, and personal questions in the meantime. What does it mean for individuals to live under conditions that place them outside the usual criteria used to describe humanness? How does society (not to mention the caregivers who are bearing witness to the human decline) sustain the course, and particularly the protracted last days, of such a disastrous condition?

Perhaps more difficult than dealing with the physical aspects of human disease and disorder is the struggle with different definitions of correct moral behavior. How are moral principles learned and sustained? How do we separate the moral from the immoral? To what extent are the definitions of moral behavior relative to socioeconomic status?

Who or what is the proper moral authority, anyway? The individual? The state? Religious institutions or leaders? The delegation of authority to any one of these has its dangers, ranging from Hemingway's formulation that "what is moral is what you feel good after," to a compromise promoted by the state such as "the greatest happiness of the greatest number," a concept that evolved from the utilitarian philosophy of Jeremy Bentham and that may have a negative impact on members of any minority in that state. But perhaps the greatest danger of all is to be found in the intersection of economics and ethical behavior, such as when, for economic reasons, battlefield triage is operative in peacetime, and only those least disabled and allegedly most likely to survive are cared for.

There are no easy answers to these questions, which are considered in this fine book, along with other topics such as physician-assisted suicide, financing long-term care, the inner experience of being demented, caregiving, advance directives, policy and decision-making, and others. Collectively, the writings in this book and their distinguished authors have made an enormous contribution. The words in the title *Dementia and Aging: Ethics, Values, and Policy Choices* are in the right order: discussion of aging and dementia creates the need to consider ethics, values, and the ultimate choices for action, since policy choices will have to be made, like it or not.

This book, then, deals with some major questions of Western civilization as they bear on the dementias, especially Alzheimer's disease, which Lewis Thomas called "the disease of the century." Even if we suddenly gained the ability to prevent the dementias and bring about even partial cures, there would still be large numbers of surviving patients with these disorders who would require our thoughts and actions for years to come.

—ROBERT N. BUTLER, M.D.
Brookdale Professor of Geriatrics and Adult Development
Chairman, Department of Geriatrics and Adult Development
The Mount Sinai Medical Center

PREFACE

It is imperative that we begin to focus attention on the ethical, moral, and policy issues raised by the growing numbers of elderly people with dementia. Already, today, some 3 million to 4 million Americans are victims of dementia. It is estimated that by the mid-twenty-first century this total will quadruple, and as many as 14 million persons may be caught up in the downward spiral of irreversible dementia, and along with them, their families and friends.

Our society must begin the challenging process of thinking through, and resolving, a number of troublesome issues that are generated by dementia. Among them are:

- How is dementia experienced by its victims? What bearing might knowledge of the experiences of persons with dementia have on the ethical and moral lights in which we see them?

- How do we perceive victims of dementia as moral beings? What bearing do these perceptions have on our sense of moral obligations toward them?

- Who should care for persons with dementia, families or society?

- What kinds of life-prolonging medical intervention are morally fitting at the various stages of dementia? When, if ever, are only care and palliation (with no intention of life prolongation) appropriate?

- Are advance directives, such as a living will and durable power of attorney, particularly useful for victims of dementia?

- Are assisted suicide and mercy killing acceptable with respect to severely demented persons, as alternatives to suffering, gradual decline, and loss of self?

- What public policies and organizational arrangements are now in place to serve victims of dementia and their families? Are they adequate? Can we afford appropriate care for persons with dementia?

- As greater amounts of financial resources are needed to cope with the high prevalence of dementia, how might they be justly allocated among research on dementia, medical intervention to save the lives of dementia patients, and long-term care and palliation for victims of dementia?

The chapters in this volume provide information, ideas, and arguments that are good starting points for facing up to such issues. The authors represent a wide range of professional and scholarly disciplines—ethics, law, medicine, nursing, philosophy, religion, political science, psychiatry, and psychology. Although their backgrounds and viewpoints are disparate, they share the conviction that it is time for us to struggle actively with the ethical, moral, and policy dilemmas posed by dementia.

Laypersons can find this book to be helpful as they confront the harsh challenges of coping with dementia as it afflicts the lives of their loved ones. Each chapter is intended for a broad audience that is interested in the personal, familial, and societal issues posed by dementia and the care of its victims. Professionals and students in virtually any clinical or scholarly field will also find that it outlines important challenges for the practical and intellectual undertakings that engage them.

In creating the plan for this book, we benefited from a series of seminars that were collaboratively sponsored by the Alzheimer Center of University Hospitals of Cleveland and the Center for Biomedical Ethics, School of Medicine, Case Western Reserve University. In producing the volume, our fellow contributors were exemplary in the quality of their work, their sense of professional responsibility, and their collegiality.

We also had support and assistance from a number of organizations and individuals. As we acknowledge them, we also express our appreciation.

Grant assistance was provided by the Cleveland Foundation, Clinical Health Laboratories of Cleveland, Gliatech Inc., Frank Greisinger, Jack Lang, Squibb Institute for Medical Research, and Warner-Lambert/Parke Davis, Inc. Case Western Reserve University contributed some faculty time and assisted with indirect expenses. Staff effort and logistic support were also provided by the Alzheimer's Association

(Cleveland chapter), the Western Reserve Geriatric Education Center, and the Center on Aging and Health of Case Western Reserve University. Marcia Bram provided the high-quality and loyal secretarial assistance that is essential to projects of this nature. Our family members were supportive in understanding the values and priorities that engaged us in this undertaking.

LIST OF CONTRIBUTORS

MARGARET P. BATTIN, Ph.D., is professor of philosophy and adjunct professor of internal medicine, Division of Medical Ethics, University of Utah. She is the author of *Ethical Issues in Suicide* (1982) and co-author or co-editor of seven other books, among them an edition of John Donne's treatise *Biathanatos*, a collection on age rationing of medical care, a casebook in aesthetics, a text on professional ethics, and a study of ethical issues in organized religion. In recent years she has been engaged in research on active euthanasia and assisted suicide in the Netherlands and Germany.

ROBERT H. BINSTOCK, Ph.D., is the Henry R. Luce Professor of Aging, Health, and Society at Case Western Reserve University, School of Medicine, Cleveland, Ohio. A former president of the Gerontological Society of America (1975–76), he has served as the director of a White House Task Force on Older Americans (1967–68) and as chair and member of many advisory panels to governments and foundations. Among his seventeen authored and edited books is *Too Old for Health Care?: Controversies in Medicine, Law, Economics, and Ethics* (1991), co-edited with Stephen G. Post.

DANIEL CALLAHAN, Ph.D., is director and co-founder of the Hastings Center, Briarcliff Manor, New York. He is an elected member of the Institute of Medicine, National Academy of Sciences; a member of the advisory council of the Office of Scientific Integrity, Department of Health and Human Services; and a member of the advisory board of the Harvard Graduate Society. He is the author or editor of thirty books, most recently including *What Kind of Life: The Limits of Medical Progress* (1990) and *Setting Limits: Medical Goals in an Aging Society* (1987).

GENE D. COHEN, M.D., Ph.D., is acting director of the National Institute on Aging (NIA), National Institutes of Health. In addition, he serves as executive secretary for both the U.S. Department of Health and Human Services Council on Alzheimer's Disease and the congressionally appointed Advisory Panel on Alzheimer's Disease. Before coming to NIA as deputy director, Dr. Cohen had served as the first chief of the Center on Aging of the National Institute of Mental Health. A former chair of the Clinical Medicine Section of the Gerontological Society of America, Dr. Cohen is editor in chief of *International Psychogeriatrics* (the journal of the International Psychogeriatric Association) and the author of a number of publications in the field of aging, including his book *The Brain in Human Aging* (1989).

REBECCA S. DRESSER, J.D., has a joint appointment as professor in the School of Law and the Center for Biomedical Ethics, School of Medicine, Case Western Reserve University. She has taught in the law and bioethics area for nine years and is the author of numerous articles in law and medical journals. She is particularly interested in issues concerning life-sustaining treatment for incompetent patients and the use of advance directives to resolve such issues.

JOSEPH M. FOLEY, M.D., is professor emeritus of neurology at the School of Medicine, Case Western Reserve University. A past president of the American Academy of Neurology, and of the American Neurological Association, he is currently chair of the Canadian Sciences Study of Alzheimer's Disease and serves on the board of directors for the Fairhill Institute for the Elderly, in Cleveland, Ohio. A pioneer in the clinical care of patients with dementia, Dr. Foley is one of the nation's leading experts in the field. In the mid-1970s he developed the first support group for the families of patients with Alzheimer's disease. His colleagues at University Hospitals of Cleveland have named their geriatric clinical facility the Joseph M. Foley Elderhealth Center.

RICHARD J. MARTIN, N.D., R.N., is an assistant professor of gerontological nursing at the Frances Payne Bolton School of Nursing, Case Western Reserve University. Dr. Martin is the assistant director for research operations at the Alzheimer Center, University Hospitals of Cleveland. He is a member of the University Hospitals of Cleveland Institutional Review Board and a charter member of the Bioethics Network of Ohio. He is currently a Commonwealth Fund Executive Nurse Fellow, studying at the Weatherhead School of Management, Case Western Reserve University.

HARRY R. MOODY, Ph.D., is deputy director of the Brookdale Center on Aging of Hunter College and is currently director of the Administration on Aging's National Eldercare Institute on Human Resources. Originally trained in the history of philosophy, he has been active in policy analysis and biomedical ethics. Moody is the author of more than sixty articles and two books—*Abundance of Life: Human Development Policies for an Aging Society* (1988) and *Ethics and Aging* (1992).

THOMAS H. MURRAY, Ph.D., is professor of biomedical ethics and director of the Center for Biomedical Ethics in the School of Medicine, Case Western Reserve University. Dr. Murray's research interests cover a wide range of ethical issues in medicine and science, including genetics, aging, children, and health policy. He is a founding editor of the journal *Medical Humanities Review* and is on the editorial boards of *Social Science and Medicine* and *Physician and Sportsmedicine*. He is an elected fellow of the Hastings Center and the Environmental Health Institute. He serves as a member of the U.S. Olympic Committee's Committee on Substance Abuse Research and Education and is a member of the Working Group on Ethical, Legal, and Social Issues, the National Institutes of Health Center for Human Genome Research. Dr. Murray has testified before congressional committees, worked often with the Office of Technology Assessment, U.S. Congress, and is the author of more than a hundred publications.

STEPHEN G. POST, Ph.D., is associate professor of biomedical ethics, School of Medicine, Case Western Reserve University. He serves as associate editor of the *Encyclopedia of Bioethics* (revised edition, 1993) and is a vice president of the Bioethics Network of Ohio. Post is a research fellow of the Kennedy Institute of Ethics, Georgetown University, and chair of the Religion, Health, and Medical Ethics section of the American Academy of Religion. The author of numerous articles on aging and ethics in journals such as the *Gerontologist* and the *Journal of the American Geriatrics Society*, Post recently co-edited, with Robert H. Binstock, a book entitled *Too Old for Health Care?: Controversies in Medicine, Law, Economics, and Ethics* (1991).

DAVID H. SMITH is director of the Poynter Center for the Study of Ethics and American Institutions, and professor of religious studies at Indiana University. He is the author of *Health and Medicine in the Anglican Tradition* (1986) and *The Achievement of John C. Bennett* (1970). He is the editor of *No Rush to Judgment: Respect and Care in Medical Ethics* (1977) and (with James T. Johnson) *Love and Society: Essays in the Ethics of Paul Ramsey* (1974).

DAVID C. THOMASMA, Ph.D., is the Michael I. English Professor of Medical Ethics and director of the Medical Humanities Program at Loyola University Chicago Medical Center, and also chief of the Ethics Consult Service and a member of the Hospital Ethics Committee. He has served on the Technical Advisory Panel for Biomedical Ethics of the American Hospital Association, and on the Theology and Ethics Advisory Committee for the Catholic Health Association. He is editor in chief of *Theoretical Medicine*, co-editor of *Cambridge Quarterly for Healthcare Ethics*, and section editor of the *Journal of the American Geriatrics Society* and serves on the editorial boards of four other journals. He has published more than 175 articles and twelve books. His most recent books are, with John Monagle, *Medical Ethics: A Guide for Health Professionals* (1988); with Edmund Pellegrino, *For the Patient's Good* (1988) and *Health and Healing Continuum* (1991); with Glenn Graber, *Theory and Practice in Medical Ethics* (1989) and *Euthanasia: Toward an Ethical Social Policy* (1990); and *Human Life in the Balance* (1990).

PETER J. WHITEHOUSE, M.D., Ph.D., is associate professor of neurology and chief of the Division of Behavioral Neurology at Case Western Reserve University. He is also director of the Alzheimer Center at University Hospitals of Cleveland, which has been designated as an Alzheimer Center of Excellence by the National Institute on Aging, the National Institute of Mental Health, and the Ohio Department on Aging. His research interests lie in the biological and clinical aspects of Alzheimer's disease and related dementias, and in health care delivery—areas in which he has published extensively. He is active in such organizations as the National Alzheimer's Association and serves as chair of the Governor's Task Force on Alzheimer's Disease for the state of Ohio.

DEMENTIA AND AGING

THE CHALLENGES
OF
DEMENTIA

Robert H. Binstock

Stephen G. Post

Peter J. Whitehouse

The attention paid to dementia, especially to Alzheimer's disease, its most common cause, has increased remarkably in the United States over the past fifteen years. A social movement, based upon alliances among scientists, caregivers of persons with dementias, government administrators, the media, and members of the general public and Congress, has transformed Alzheimer's disease from "an obscure, rarely applied medical diagnosis to [a] characterization as the fourth or fifth leading cause of death in the United States" (Fox, 1989, p. 58). Federal funding of biomedical research on Alzheimer's disease increased from less than $4 million in 1976 to $140 million in 1990 (Office of Technology Assessment, 1990, p. 8).

THE NATURE AND EXTENT OF DEMENTIA

Dementia, a global cognitive syndrome caused by diseases acquired in adulthood, poses enormous challenges to patients, family members, clinicians, health care policymakers, and scientists. The diseases that cause dementia bring about a disruption of an individual's sense of personal history by impairing memory, and later progress to impair other intellectual faculties such as language and perception; eventually the patient loses even the ability to understand his or her own plight and is completely dependent on others to care for all basic bodily functions. Family members find themselves dealing with a disorder that robs their loved one of individuality and autonomy, yet leaves the physical self intact. The clinician is hampered by the absence of specific therapies and specific diagnostic tests for the more common conditions such as Alzheimer's disease, and even by a lack of sufficient knowledge of normal cognition to provide a frame of reference for understanding dementia. Health care policymakers are daunted by their recognition that dementia is an epidemic that reveals dramatically the failure of our health care system to deal with chronic illnesss and disability. And dementia challenges biomedical researchers to understand how genes and environment regulate aging, how nerve cells function and fail to function, and how human behavior is dependent on interconnected neural systems.

The challenges posed by Alzheimer's disease and other causes of dementia will increase dramatically in the future. Today, an estimated 4 million Americans suffer from dementia; 55 percent of them are so severely incapacitated that they require continuous care. The prevalence of dementia increases with age, from less than 1 percent of persons under age 65, to about 1 percent of those aged 65 to 74, 7 percent of those 75 to 84, and 25 percent of those aged 85 and older (Office of Technology Assessment, 1990, p. 11). When we consider that the number of Americans reaching the older old-age categories is increasing substantially, it is highly likely that the number of victims of dementia will grow substantially in the decades ahead. In 1990, for instance, there were 3.3 million persons aged 85 and older, constituting 10 percent of the population aged 65 and older; in the year 2000 there will be 4.6 million, or 13 percent; and by 2040 some 12.3 million persons aged 85 and older will account for 18 percent of the elderly population (Taeuber, 1990, p. 3). One estimate (Schneider and Guralnik, 1990) suggests that the number of severely and moderately demented patients will quadruple by 2040, requiring a more than fourfold increase in health care expenditures on such patients from $35.8 billion in 1985 to as much as $149 billion (in 1985 dollars). Similar concerns about a growing epidemic of dementia within older populations have been expressed in Japan and other developed nations that are experiencing rapid population aging (Martin, 1989).

Some dementias are reversible, for example those due to metabolic dysfunction in the body, such as hypothyroidism, or those due to surgically treatable structural lesions of the brain, such as benign tumors. But reversible dementias are rare. The most common forms of dementia—those caused by Alzheimer's and other degenerative diseases, such as Parkinson's, Huntington's, and Pick's—tend to be irreversible and progressive (see chapter 2). An ongoing investment in basic biomedical research is needed to find ways to cure these forms of dementia.

CARING FOR PEOPLE WITH DEMENTIA

Although research on the causes of dementias has progressed somewhat in the past few years (see Goate et al., 1991; Kolata, 1991), the development of effective ways to prevent and cure dementias is not likely in the years immediately ahead (Office of Technology Assessment, 1987). Therapies that offer symptomatic treatment or slow the progress of dementia might be available soon. But even at present, humane modes of care and services can be provided, both to lessen the suffering of people who are afflicted with irreversible dementia, and to reduce the physical, emotional, and financial burdens of families and others who provide care for these patients.

A large range of medical, nursing, social, legal, financial, and other long-term care services that can be of value to dementia patients and their caregivers have been identified through program development and research (see table 1). Although each of these types of services tends to be used as well for long-term care patients with other forms of disease and disability, the cognitive impairments of people with dementia often require that the nature of the service be altered. A prime reason for this is that a demented patient often fails to understand and cooperate with service providers; by the same token, many service providers are not especially knowledgeable about or skilled at working with patients who have dementia. Because of such differences some advocates for demented patients and their families have urged the development of a separate *dementia-specific* service system. Others argue that a broader, generic service system is sufficient if it can be *dementia-capable*, that is, effective in working with dementia patients and their caregivers and knowledgeable about the kinds of services that may be especially helpful (see Office of Technology Assessment, 1990, p. 33).

Whether a dementia patient is living at home, in a nursing home, or in another type of residential setting, an ideal system of services would be amply available, of high quality, provided by well-trained personnel, easily located and arranged, and well funded through public and private resources. The present system, however, is far from ideal.

The supply of services is insufficient; service providers lack education and training; and the quality of many services is poor (Office of Technology Assessment, 1987). Moreover, the system is so fragmented that even when high-quality services are sufficiently available, many patients and families do not know about them and require help in defining their service needs and in arranging for them to be provided (Office of Technology Assessment, 1990).

Underlying each of these problems, in turn, is the issue of financing.

TABLE 1.

Services That May Be Needed for People with Dementia and Their Families

Diagnosis	Protective services
Acute medical care	Supervision
Ongoing medical supervision	Home health aide
Treatment of coexisting medical conditions	Homemaker
Medication and elimination of drugs that cause excess disability	Personal care
	Paid companion/sitter
	Shopping
Multidimensional assessment	Home-delivered meals
Skilled nursing	Chore services
Physical therapy	Telephone reassurance
Occupational therapy	Personal emergency response system
Speech therapy	Recreation/exercise
Adult day care	Transportation
Respite care*	Escort service
Family/caregiver education and training	Special equipment (ramps, hospital beds, etc.)
Family/caregiver counseling	Vision care
Family support groups	Audiology
Patient counseling	Dental care
Legal services	Nutrition counseling
Financial/benefits counseling	Hospice
Mental health services	Autopsy

Source: Office of Technology Assessment, 1990, p. 16.

Note: Most of these services may be needed by and can be provided for patients who are living at home, in a nursing home, or in another residential care facility, such as a board and care facility, adult foster home, or sheltered housing.

Respite care includes any service intended to provide temporary relief for the primary caregiver. When used for that purpose, homemaker, paid companion/sitter, adult day care, temporary nursing home care, and other services included on the list constitute respite care.

As is the case with most aspects of the U.S. health care delivery system, the characteristics of long-term care services are substantially shaped by the nature and extent of policies for funding it (see Hudson, 1990; Kane and Kane, 1990). Accordingly, success in reforming long-term care services, to make them both adequate in supply and appropriate in quality and accessibility, will largely lie in efforts to change the nature of funding them.

CONSTITUENCIES AND COSTS FOR LONG-TERM CARE REFORM

The service needs of dementia patients and their families are inextricably linked with the overlapping and parallel needs encountered by any of us—regardless of illness, disability, family situation, or age—who are faced with issues of long-term care. The essentiality of this linkage is manifest in the recent report of a national panel of experts which, though convened to consider the problems faced in locating and arranging appropriate services for people with dementia, recommended overwhelmingly that Congress enact solutions that "serve people with dementia and people with other conditions and diseases as well" (Office of Technology Assessment, 1990, p. 63). It is likely that any major governmental action to expand, improve, and make more accessible the services that help dementia patients and their families will be incorporated in broader initiatives for reforming and financing long-term care in the United States.

THE CONSTITUENCIES

Substantial public recognition of a need to reform long-term care is relatively recent. Some of the increased awareness can be traced directly to successful advocacy efforts that have focused on dementias, particularly Alzheimer's disease (Fox, 1989).

At the forefront of such efforts has been the national Alzheimer's Association, based in Chicago and Washington, and its 200 chapters in forty-nine states. A voluntary association founded in 1980—comprising families, researchers, health care professionals, and service providers—it has five primary goals:

- to support research in the cause, treatment, cure, and prevention of Alzheimer's disease and related disorders;

- to stimulate awareness of Alzheimer's disease among the public and professionals;

- to encourage the formation of Alzheimer's Association chapters to create a nationwide support network for families of people with Alzheimer's disease;

- to advocate for Federal, State, and local public policies and legislation to assist Alzheimer's patients and their families;

- and to provide community programs and services for people with Alzheimer's disease and their families. (Alzheimer's Association, 1987)

Also important in the evolution of demands for reforming long-term care has been a growing constituency of adult children of elderly patients who are perceiving the importance of long-term care services because of their direct contact with the experiences and issues of providing or arranging for the care of their aged parents afflicted by any one or more of a wide variety of disabilities and diseases (Brody, 1985,

1990). More than 13 million adults in the United States who have disabled elderly parents or spouses are potential providers of long-term care, financial assistance, and emotional support; 4.2 million of them currently provide direct care in home settings (Stone and Kemper, 1989). Nursing home care is provided to another 1.4 million persons daily (Lazenby and Letsch, 1990).

The mutual concerns and interests of advocates for victims of dementia and for the broader constituency concerned with chronically ill and disabled older persons are more than an intellectual abstraction. They have been directly acknowledged and expressed since 1988 when the Alzheimer's Association, the American Association for Retired Persons (AARP), and the Villers Foundation (a small organization focused on the plight of poor older people) allied to undertake a lobbying effort organized formally as Long-Term Care '88 during the 1988 presidential campaign (McConnell, 1990).

Disabled children, younger disabled adults, and their families, respectively, are additional potential constituencies to support greater development of long-term care. In the context of ubiquitous discussions regarding the "health care needs of an aging society" (e.g., Committee on an Aging Society, 1985), it is important to note, for instance, that the number of functionally disabled adults aged 18 to 64 years who live outside institutions is more than twice the total of all comparably disabled persons aged 65 and older (Gornick et al., 1985, pp. 22–23). Some leaders of organizations representing disabled people (Rubenfeld, 1986) and older people (Torres-Gil, in press) have expressed the hope that a coalition of organizations representing disabled and older people, and their families, will be developed as a powerful force in American politics.

As an expression of this broad range of potential constituencies the lobbying efforts for long-term care which were launched in the 1988 presidential campaign have been carried forward by a coalition named The Long-Term Care Campaign. This Washington-based interest group claims to represent nearly 140 national organizations (with more than 60 million members) including religious denominations; organized labor and business groups; nurses, veterans, youth, and women groups; consumer organizations; and racial and ethnic groups, as well as older persons. Among its key legislative objectives are:

- Long-Term Care services should be available to all who need them, regardless of age or income.

- A national Long-Term Care program should provide a comprehensive range of facility-based and community-based health, social and supportive services to maintain and enhance personal independence. (Long-Term Care Campaign, 1990)

THE COSTS

Paying the costs of long-term care can be a catastrophic financial experience for patients and their families. For instance, five years ago a congressional report estimated that such care for a victim of Alzheimer's disease can cost from $25,000 to $65,000 annually (U.S. House of Representatives, 1987). Undoubtedly, the range of costs is substantially higher today.

More than eighty federal programs, and a plethora of state and local public and private agencies, are sources of funding for services needed by dementia patients (Congressional Research Service, 1988). But each source regulates the availability of funds with rules as to eligibility and breadth of service coverage, and changes its rules frequently. Dementia patients are often ruled ineligible for funding through Medicare, Medicaid, and other programs (Office of Technology Assessment, 1987). Thus, despite the many sources of funding, specific patients and caregivers may find themselves ineligible for financial help and unable to pay out of pocket for needed services. In one study about 75 percent of the caregivers for dementia patients reported that they did not use services because they were unable to pay for them (Eckert and Smyth, 1988).

The annual cost of a year's care in a nursing home averages $25,000 (U.S. General Accounting Office, 1989, p. 34) and ranges as high as $80,000. Equivalent care provided in a home setting is just as expensive when the in-kind, informal services provided by family and friends of a patient are included as expenses. Although nursing homes originally developed as an alternative to home care, their financial costs have redirected great attention during the past two decades to home care as a possible cheaper alternative. But numerous demonstrations and studies have concluded that home care is not a cost-effective substitute for nursing home care (Kane and Kane, 1987; Weissert, 1990).

Patients and their families paid more than $22 billion out of pocket for long-term care services in 1989. The total national expenditure for long-term care was an estimated $60 billion. Expenditures on nursing homes were $47.9 billion; home care services provided by agencies participating in Medicare and Medicaid accounted for $6.6 billion. Payments to other home care service providers accounted for an estimated $5.5 billion in additional expenditures.* Out-of-pocket pay-

*This estimate is calculated by assuming that nursing home payments were 80 percent of the national total of long-term care expenditures, as reported by the U.S. General Accounting Office (1989, p. 31) for the fiscal year 1985.

ments accounted for 44 percent of all nursing home expenditures and 11 percent of home care expenditures (Lazenby and Letsch, 1990, pp. 4–8).

The Medicare health insurance program does not reimburse patients for long-term care, either in nursing homes or at home. Private long-term care insurance, in an early stage of product development, is very expensive for the majority of persons, and its benefits are limited in scope and duration. Only 3 percent of older persons have any private long-term care insurance, and only about 1 percent of nursing home costs are paid for by private insurance (Wiener, 1990). Even when the product matures, it is unlikely to be a panacea. A Brookings Institution study suggested that by the year 2018, when all the "bugs" are worked out, some 25 percent to 45 percent of elderly people would be able to afford private long-term care insurance premiums, and that private insurance benefit payments would only account for 7 to 12 percent of all nursing home benefits (Rivlin and Wiener, 1988).

Medicaid, the federal-state insurance program available to persons of all ages who qualify through classification as economically poor, does pay for long-term care in nursing homes (accounting for nearly 50 percent of total national nursing home expenditures). But Medicaid does not pay for the full range of home care services that will be needed in most cases. Most state Medicaid programs provide reimbursement only for the most "medicalized" services that are necessary to maintain a long-term care patient in a home environment; rarely reimbursed are essential supports such as chore services, assistance with food shopping and meal preparation, transportation, companionship, periodic monitoring, and respite programs for family and other unpaid caregivers. Medicaid does include a special waiver program that allows states to offer a wider range of nonmedical home care services, if limited to those patients who otherwise would require Medicaid-financed nursing home care. Although forty-two states participate in this waiver program, relatively few dependent patients are helped. The National Governors Association estimated that only 59,000 elderly persons were served by the waiver program in 1987 (U.S. General Accounting Office, 1989, p. 27).

As an alternative to public and private insurance coverage for the full range of formal home care services, many have looked to the family as a source for informal, unpaid supportive care. But it is estimated that about 85 percent of the various elements of the continuum of care necessary for living in the community is currently provided by family members on a voluntary basis (U.S. Senate, 1989). Of those dependent older persons who receive care, an overwhelming majority receive such informal care. About 74 percent receive all their care from family members or other unpaid sources; about 21 percent receive both formal and informal services; and only about 5 percent use formal, paid services exclusively (Liu et al., 1985, p. 52).

There is no basis for expecting that families can be looked to as an even greater source of in-kind financing that will meet the growing need for long-term care as our population ages. In fact, demographic trends, changing patterns of family structure, and a persistent upward trend in labor force participation by middle-aged women who have traditionally provided much of this care suggest that the current rate of informal caregiving could even decline (see Brody, 1990; U.S. General Accounting Office, 1989).

Even in this present context of substantial informal care, complemented by an additional $60 billion in purchased, formal services, persons with long-term disabilities and disease do not get all the supportive assistance that they require. An analysis from the 1982 National Long-Term Care Survey showed that 40 percent of dependent older Americans were not receiving all of the help they needed with activities of daily living which ranged from getting in and out of bed to getting around outside the home (Stone et al., 1987).

Expanding home care services to meet such unmet needs, and providing public insurance coverage for the $22 billion that patients and their families pay out of pocket for services, have been the central objectives of several dozen recent congressional proposals to reform long-term care (Wiener, 1990). A half dozen major bills introduced in Congress have also responded to a wide range of the constituencies interested in reforming long-term care, by taking broad approaches to defining the populations of patients which would be eligible for coverage. Many of these bills have defined patient eligibility to include either disabled children or disabled adults under age 65, or both, as well as all disabled persons aged 65 and older.

Reflecting these ambitious approaches, the estimated costs of the major proposals for reforming long-term care which were introduced in the 100th Congress were substantial, ranging from $21 billion to $50 billion in projected expenditures for the first year (OMB Watch, 1990, p. 18). The large range in estimated costs is due to variations among the proposals regarding specific populations eligible for coverage, as well as differences in technical provisions regarding the timing, nature, and extent of insurance coverage.

Because any major public long-term care initiative is expected to cost tens of billions of dollars, most analysts of congressional health policies and politics do not expect such a reform to be enacted within the next few years. In the present political context the public resources available for such a purpose are perceived as scarce. The need to "reduce the deficit" is a rhetorical mainstay of domestic politics. "Containing health care costs" is widely considered to be one of the major goals of our society. Moreover, the relatively recent poltical experiences of enacting the Medicare Catastrophic Coverage Act in 1988 and repealing it in 1989 (discussed in chapter 11) have made some members of Congress particularly wary of undertaking a major expansion of health care benefits that centrally involve older persons (Atkins, 1990; Crystal, 1990; Wiener, 1990).

Ironically, just when the principle of expanding public long-term care insurance is favored by many leaders in Congress, the economic costs of doing so appear to be politically prohibitive. In 1990, for example, a long-awaited report of the U.S. Bipartisan Commission on Comprehensive Health Care (also known as the Pepper Commission) boldly recommended a program of long-term care services for any American who needs them, with an annual cost of $43 billion. But because the commission did not identify a source of funds for paying the $43 billion, the report had little impact. As the chairman of the health subcommittee of the House Ways and Means Committee put it, "Without a way to pay for it, it is a non-starter. It is legislatively dead" (Tolchin, 1990, p. 1).

In short, although proposals to reform and publicly fund long-term care are now firmly on the public policy agenda, their adoption and implementation may be some years off. Today, in the early 1990s, adequate development of humane modes of care and services for dementia patients remains a major challenge along with the challenges of identifying the causes of dementias, preventing them, and treating and curing them.

AN OVERVIEW OF THE VOLUME

The chapters in this volume are arranged so as to follow the chronology of dementia from the experience of those who are afflicted by it at its earliest stages, through the moral challenges of caregiving, treatment decisions, euthanasia, and public policy. The authors represent a wide range of professions and disciplines, conveying broad scientific and humanistic perspectives on the moral and policy issues addressed.

Part 1, "Biomedical, Experiential, and Caregiving Perspectives," presents humanistic interpretations of dementia as experienced by its victims, by family members, and by caregivers. In chapter 2, "Dementia: The Medical Perspective," Peter J. Whitehouse, M.D., Ph.D., a neurologist and psychologist, summarizes the clinical and biological aspects of dementia, distinguishing between degenerative diseases such as Alzheimer's, multi-infarct dementias, and other forms of dementing illnesses. Whitehouse focuses especially on the clinical features of Alzheimer's disease, beginning with amnesia and progressing to dependence in activities of daily living, including the inability to eat. Behavioral changes, from early affective symptoms to frank psychosis, are briefly described; the biological bases of Alzheimer's disease, including recent genetic hypotheses, are examined. Whitehouse concludes with an overview of research issues for the future. Biologically, the most critical questions are: What causes Alzheimer's disease? Why do nerve cells die? Which ones die? Clinical research on these issues is progressing, and in the years immediately ahead experiments will be conducted to see if medications are useful.

In the third chapter, "The Experience of Being Demented," Joseph M. Foley, M.D., a pioneer in the study of neurology and dementia, is concerned with dementia as the sufferer experiences it. He relies in part on an interview with an elderly man recently diagnosed as having probable Alzheimer's disease. Foley interprets the words and feelings of the sufferer, who was sufficiently competent to consent to the interview. In particular, Foley treats the ways in which the sufferer might attempt to compensate for his loss of memory throughout the conversation. He also emphasizes the anxieties experienced by the sufferer, and the stages of anxiety related to the progress of Alzheimer's disease generally. Through this chapter, one is able to understand and empathize with the struggles of those who are only mildly demented but are very much aware of their gradual decline. Foley emphasizes that caregivers must have an awareness of the insights and feelings of demented patients.

The focus in the fourth chapter shifts from dementia as experienced by patients to dementia as others perceive it. David H. Smith, Ph.D., a biomedical ethicist, reflects poignantly on his own family's response to the gradual decline of his mother-in-law. In his chapter, "Seeing and Knowing Dementia," Smith argues against the view that persons who lose much of their self-identity and their cognition to dementia are no longer entitled to the same level of loyalty as those who are cognitively intact. Underlying the diminishment of demented people is the potentially dangerous cultural assumption that persons who are no longer productive and fully rational are worthless. Smith criticizes some of the negative metaphors and analogies that are occasionally applied to demented persons. Much of his analysis is existential, focusing on how the demented person confronts us with an image of human deterioration which we would prefer to avoid, and therefore ridicule. Smith counsels loyalty, compassion, and a recognition of shortcomings in some of the ethical theories that bear on these values.

Richard J. Martin, D.N., a nurse, and Stephen G. Post, Ph.D., an ethicist, deal with the theme of direct caregiving for the demented elderly person. In chapter 5, "Human Dignity, Dementia, and the Moral Basis of Caregiving," they consider the moral basis for caregiving within both the family and institutions, as well as the moral challenges of what some interpret as demeaning caregiver tasks. The perspective of the nursing profession is combined with ideas about caring which are gleaned from philosophy and religious thought. Martin and Post stress the importance of the virtue of care in medical ethics and note the overemphasis on difficult life-and-death decisions in recent medical-ethics literature. In particular, they give consideration to the caregiving "women in the middle" (see Brody, 1990) and the strains of filial duties which affect daughter and daughter-in-law.

Perspectives on the experience of dementia, as provided by the four chapters in part 1, form a context for part 2, "Treatment Decisions, Advance Directives, and Euthanasia." The chapters in this section focus on the difficult decisions surrounding the end of life.

Rebecca S. Dresser, J.D., a lawyer and ethicist, evaluates advance directives (such as living wills), legal instruments that attempt to anticipate decisions on behalf of patients who are not mentally competent. In chapter 6, "Autonomy Revisited: The Limits of Anticipatory Choices," she argues that treatment decisions should be more explicitly focused on the incompetent patient's current best interests, rather than on what the patient might have wished while still competent. The competent person's prior designation of his or her treatment preferences through advance directives is less morally compelling than the incompetent patient's interest in protection from substantial harm. Limits on "precedent autonomy" are necessary for society to maintain its moral concern for vulnerable, disabled individuals. Dresser does think that advance directives are generally useful, but she casts doubt on their value in the context of the long decline associated with dementia.

Harry R. Moody, Ph.D., a philosopher, also addresses the issues of advance directives and treatment decisions. In chapter 7, "A Critical View of Ethical Dilemmas in Dementia," Moody sees advance directives as largely symbolic expressions of a communication process that is ongoing and constantly open to revision. Each stage of dementia involves renegotiating goals, expectations, and obligations as the patient's condition changes. This requires continuing dialogue between health care providers and family members who will generally be deeply invested in decision-making. No piece of paper will allow an escape from the ongoing challenge of communication and negotiation. Advance directives do have a place in the process of communication, offering valuable information about a patient's preferences. But, concludes Moody, they are most useful as an occasion for broaching value questions among patient, family, and health care providers, before the onset of dementia. It is from this model of negotiation and communication between all "legitimate stakeholders," he feels, that progress will emerge.

While both Moody and Dresser support some use of advance directives, they do not regard such instruments as morally compelling in all cases. Although worthwhile, they are not a substitute for wider negotiations or for decisions consistent with the good of the severely demented patient.

The eighth and ninth chapters, on euthanasia (mercy killing) of demented elderly people, represent distinctive frameworks. Humanist David C. Thomasma, Ph.D., while not ruling out euthanasia in certain rare and unusual cases, prefers to prohibit the practice and to encourage modern medicine to work harder in research areas that promise to make the dying process as comfortable as possible. His chapter, "Mercy Killing of Elderly People with Dementia: A Counterproposal," underscores alternatives to active euthanasia. Dementia and euthanasia have been intertwined in much recent debate, and euthanasia policies such as those existing in the Netherlands (Have, 1989) have a particular impact on the elderly patient. In contrast to those who favor preemptive suicide (e.g., Prado, 1990), Thomasma is decidedly conserving of basic moral restraints against killing. He does favor passive euthanasia—that is, withholding or withdrawing medical technology—as an appropriate response to the sufferings of patients.

Margaret P. Battin, Ph.D., a philosopher, develops a different line of argument in her chapter, "Euthanasia in Alzheimer's Disease?" She shows how difficult questions of euthanasia become when applied to demented persons. She focuses strictly on "direct killing, performed in the paradigmatic case by a physician as a medical procedure intended to produce death." As Battin reviews arguments for euthanasia which might be derived from reference to principles of autonomy, mercy, and justice (expenditure of funds for care on Alzheimer's victims as a "waste"), she finds none of them fully convincing. Similarly, she is not persuaded by standard arguments against euthanasia, such as the classic "slippery slope" of moral decline. Her conclusion is: "Philosophical reflection seems to produce no compelling argument against euthanasia in advanced Alzheimer's, and no reason why we should fear it." Battin suggests active euthanasia, but *only* on the basis of an "antecedently executed living will or personal directive requesting it." This conclusion contrasts sharply with that of Thomasma.

The final part of this book, "Caring for People with Dementia: Justice and Public Policy," contains two chapters that present very different views on how to achieve appropriate care for people with dementia. In chapter 10, "Dementia and Appropriate Care: Allocating Scarce Resources," Daniel Callahan, Ph.D., a biomedical ethicist, holds that dementias deserve the highest priority in health care for elderly people because they rob sufferers of respect and dignity. However, our medical research system does not place much emphasis on personal care and social services; its focus is cure rather than care. Can we change a system that will finance coronary bypass operations for octogenarians with only a short life expectancy thereafter but that does not provide sufficient long-term care for the victims of dementia? Callahan sees a trade-off between curing and caring, since so much money is already spent on health care and it is unlikely that spending more will have public appeal. Moreover, a society needs to invest in areas other than health care, such as housing and education. "There is increasingly little reason," argues Callahan, "to continually expand resources for health care when so many other sectors are suffering even worse deprivations." Research to cure dementias should proceed, but expensive therapeutic approaches should be avoided, "because of the condition, not primarily the age, of the patient." Patients whose dementias are not far advanced might qualify for acute-care medicine, but those whose "personhood has been severely compromised" will not.

Robert H. Binstock, Ph.D., a political scientist, and Thomas H. Murray, Ph.D., a biomedical ethicist, agree with Callahan that the development of appropriate long-term care is just and essential. In sharp contrast with Callahan, however, they do not view such a development as feasible through setting limits on the use of health care resources for curing elderly people. In chapter 11, "The Politics of Developing Appropriate Care for Dementia," they maintain that even if it were ethically and morally acceptable to deny lifesaving care to older persons, it is politically naive to suggest that the financial savings that could be achieved through such rationing would be reallocated to long-term care. Moreover, they suggest that the amount of funds saved from denying expensive lifesaving care would hardly begin to fund an adequate long-term care system.

Binstock and Murray suggest that appropriate services for dementia victims and their families are most likely to be realized through an explicit and direct national policy that specifies new tax revenues to expand the public resources available for long-term care. If sufficient political support is to be developed for such a policy, they believe that an essential first step is widespread grass-roots dialogues to develop some degree of popular consensus on fundamental issues of distributive justice, such as: Why should moderately well-off and wealthy persons be protected by government from having to spend their income and assets on long-term health and social care? Which citizens might be taxed to preserve the income and assets—and ultimately the legacies—of others?

In a concluding chapter 12, "Alzheimer's Disease: Current Policy Initiatives," Gene D. Cohen, M.D., deputy director of the National Institute on Aging, describes the evolution of governmental policies and programs of research and services which deal with dementia. He underscores the complex challenges posed by dementia, pointing out the ways in which current policy deliberations appropriately reflect that complexity.

REFERENCES

Alzheimer's Association. (1987). *National Program to Conquer Alzheimer's Disease.* Chicago: Alzheimer's Disease and Related Disorders Association.

Atkins, G.L. (1990). The politics of financing long-term care. *Generations, 14*(2):19–22.

Brody, E.M. (1985). Parent care as a normative family stress. *Gerontologist, 25*:19–29.

Brody, E.M. (1990). *Women in the Middle: Their Parent-Care Years.* New York: Springer Publishing Co.

Committee on an Aging Society/Institute of Medicine and National Research Council. (1985). *Health in an Older Society.* Washington, D.C.: National Academy Press.

Congressional Research Service, Library of Congress, Congress of the United States. (1988). *Financing and Delivery of Long-Term Care Services for the Elderly.* Washington, D.C.: U.S. Government Printing Office.

Crystal, S. (1990). Health economics, old-age politics, and the Catastrophic Medicare debate. *Journal of Gerontological Social Work, 15*(3/4):21–31.

Eckert, S.K., and Smyth, K. (1988). *A Case Study of Methods of Locating and Arranging Health and Long-Term Care for Persons with Dementia.* Washington, D.C.: Office of Technology Assessment, Congress of the United States.

Fox, P. (1989). From senility to Alzheimer's disease: the rise of the Alzheimer's disease movement. *Milbank Quarterly, 67*:58–102.

Goate, A., Chartier-Harlin, M.-C., Mullan, M., Brown, J., Crawford, F., Fidani, L., Giuffra, L., Haynes, A., Irving, N., James, L., Mant, R., Newton, P., Rooke, K., Roques, P., Talbot, C., Pericak-Vance, M., Roses, A., Williamson, R., Rossor, M., Owen, M., and Hardy, J. (1991). Segregation of a missense mutation in the amyloid precursor protein gene with familial Alzheimer's disease. *Nature, 349*:704–706.

Gornick, M., Greenberg, J.N., Eggers, P.W., and Dobson, A. (1985). Twenty years of Medicare and Medicaid: covered populations, use of benefits, and program expenditures. *Health Care Financing Review, Annual Supplement:* 13–59.

Have, H.M.J. ten. (1989). Euthanasia in the Netherlands: the legal context and the cases. *Hospital Ethics Committee Forum: An Interdisciplinary Journal on Hospitals' Ethical and Legal Issues*, 1:41–45.

Hudson, R.H. (1990). Home care policy: loved by all, feared by many. In C. Zuckerman, N.N. Dubler, and B. Collopy, eds., *Home Health Care Options*, pp. 271–301. New York: Plenum Press.

Kane, R.A., and Kane, R.L. (1987). *Long-Term Care: Principles, Programs, and Policies*. New York: Springer Publishing Co.

Kane, R.L., and Kane, R.A. (1990). Health care for older people: organizational and policy issues. In R.H. Binstock and L.K. George, eds., *Handbook of Aging and the Social Sciences* (3d ed.), pp. 415–437. San Diego: Academic Press.

Kolata, G. (1991). Alzheimer's researchers close in on causes. *New York Times* (February 26):B5.

Lazenby, H.C., and Letsch, S.W. (1990). National health expenditures, 1989. *Health Care Financing Review*, 12(2):1–26.

Liu, K., Manton, K., and Liu, B.M. (1985). Home care expenses for the disabled elderly. *Health Care Financing Review*, 7:51–58.

Long-Term Care Campaign. (1990). Pepper Commission recommendations released March 2nd. *Insiders' Update* (January/February):1.

Martin, L.G. (1989). *The Graying of Japan*. Washington, D.C.: Population Reference Bureau, Inc. (Population Bulletin No. 2, July).

McConnell, S. (1990). Who cares about long-term care? *Generations*, 14(2): 15–18.

Office of Technology Assessment, Congress of the United States. (1987). *Losing a Million Minds: Confronting the Tragedy of Alzheimer's Disease and Other Dementias*. Washington, D.C.: U.S. Government Printing Office.

Office of Technology Assessment, Congress of the United States. (1990). *Confused Minds, Burdened Families: Finding Help for People with Alzheimer's and Other Dementias*. Washington, D.C.: U.S. Government Printing Office.

OMB Watch. (1990). *Long-term Care Policy: Where Are We Going?* Boston: Gerontology Institute, University of Massachusetts at Boston.

Prado, C.G. (1990). *The Last Choice: Preemptive Suicide in Advanced Age*. Westport, Conn.: Greenwood Press.

Rivlin, A.M., and Wiener, J.M. (1988). *Caring for the Disabled Elderly: Who Will Pay?* Washington, D.C.: Brookings Institution.

Rubenfeld, P. (1986). Ageism and disabilityism: double jeopardy. In S.J. Brody and G.E. Ruff, eds., *Aging and Rehabilitation: Advances in the State of the Art*, pp. 323–328. New York: Springer Publishing Co.

Schneider, E.L., and Guralnik, J.M. (1990). The aging of America: impact on health care costs. *Journal of the American Medical Association*, 263:2335–2340.

Stone, R., Cafferata, G.L., and Sangl, J. (1987). Caregivers of the frail elderly: a national profile. *Gerontologist*, 27:616–626.

Stone, R., and Kemper, P. (1989). Spouses and children of disabled elders: how large a constituency for long-term care reform? *Milbank Quarterly*, 67:485–506.

Taeuber, C. (1990). Diversity: the dramatic reality. In S. Bass, E. Kutza, and F. Torres-Gill, eds., *Diversity in Aging: Challenges facing Planners and Policymakers in the 1990s*, pp. 1–45. Glenview, Ill.: Scott, Foresman and Co.

Tolchin, M. (1990). Panel says broad health care would cost $86 billion a year. *New York Times* (March 3):1.

Torres-Gil, F.M. (In press). Interest group politics, diversity, and long-term care. In V.L. Greene and T.M. Smeeding, eds., *Social Policy for an America Growing Older.* Syracuse, N.Y.: Maxwell School For Citizenship and Public Affairs, Syracuse University.

U.S. General Accounting Office. (1989). *Long-Term Care for the Elderly: Issues of Need, Access, and Cost* (GAO/HRD-89-4). Washington, D.C.: U.S. Government Printing Office.

U.S. House of Representatives, Select Committee on Aging. (1987). *Paying the Price of Catastrophic Illness: From Accidents to Alzheimer's.* Washington, D.C.: U.S. Government Printing Office.

U.S. Senate, Special Committee on Aging. (1989). *Aging America: Trends and Projections.* Washington, D.C.: U.S. Government Printing Office.

Weissert, W.G. (1990). Strategies for reducing home care expenditures. *Generations, 14*(2):42–44.

Wiener, J.M., ed. (1990). Which way for long-term care financing? *Generations, 14*(2):4–9.

PART I. Biomedical, Experiential,
         and Caregiving Perspectives

2

DEMENTIA:
THE MEDICAL PERSPECTIVE

Peter J. Whitehouse

The exploration of the ethical and public policy implications surrounding dementia requires understanding dementia both as a medical syndrome and as a personal experience. This chapter views dementia as seen by professionals. It starts with a summary of the defining characteristics of dementia and its major causes, followed by a discussion of the clinical and biological features of the most common dementia, Alzheimer's disease (AD). The final sections focus on key research questions, which, if answered, may both aid our current debates of some ethical and public policy concerns and create new questions and concerns in their stead.

DEMENTIA

Dementia is a syndrome characterized by loss of cognitive abilities occurring in clear consciousness. Diagnostic criteria include a deterioration from a previous state of either normality or at least static cognitive ability (e.g., previously stable mental retardation). Acute changes in mental status, often associated with metabolic derangements due to systemic illnesses, are called delirium and are differentiated from dementia. Dementias can be fixed or static in time, such as the diffuse cognitive impairment that can occur in a young individual who has suffered a single episode of head trauma, or they can be progressive, such as occurs in degenerative dementias (e.g., Alzheimer's disease). Dementias can be reversible, such as those caused by endocrine dysfunction (e.g., hypothyroidism), or irreversible, if the pathophysiological process cannot be reversed and the underlying disease continues. All dementias are treatable in that professionals can provide assistance to victim and family regardless of whether a specific cure or intervention of meaningful biological magnitude is available.

THE CAUSES OF DEMENTIA

Dementia can be caused by more than fifty illnesses (Cummings and Benson, 1983). A careful medical examination is required of all individuals who suffer from cognitive difficulties. The most common causes of dementia are the degenerative dementias, such as AD, which is discussed in greater detail later in this chapter.

Degenerative dementias are conditions in which the cardinal biological feature is the loss of specific populations of neurons. These disorders usually occur in older individuals, are frequently idiopathic (i.e., they do not have a specific known cause), and are progressive (i.e., neurons continue to die and the patient's cognitive abilities deteriorate). Other degenerative dementias besides AD include the dementias associated with Parkinson's disease, Huntington's disease, Pick's disease, and a large group of rarer conditions that are hard to distinguish from AD in life. The second most common causes of dementia are multi-infarct dementia (MID) and a mixture of MID and AD. MID is a condition in which several areas of brain die because of lack of blood flow or hemorrhage, most usually due to atherosclerosis or hypertension. Patients with this condition often evidence vascular disease outside the central nervous system and frequently show a stepwise deterioration. A mixture of AD and MID is probably due to the chance occurrence, together, of two common diseases.

Compared with degenerative and vascular diseases, other conditions that cause dementia are rare. The effects of overuse of over-the-counter or prescription drugs that affect cognition can mimic dementia. Depression can cause cognitive impairment and can be confused with a neurological condition that causes progressive deterioration. Several potentially reversible dementias are those due to chronic metabolic dysfunctions and hepatic or renal failure, for example, or structural lesions in the central nervous system (CNS) such as benign tumors. In an individual with appropriate risk factors, AIDS dementia needs to be considered.

Every patient with cognitive impairment requires a history, physical examination, and laboratory tests to establish as best as possible the cause of the dementia. Screening blood tests can exclude vitamin deficiencies, endocrine abnormalities, and electrolyte imbalances. A brain imaging test, either computerized tomography (CT) or magnetic resonance imaging (MRI), is necessary to diagnose structural lesions in the central nervous system, such as tumors or subdural hematomas. CT or MRI can also provide evidence for the multiple strokes necessary to make the diagnosis of vascular dementia.

There is no specific diagnostic test for the most common dementia, AD, although brain imaging shows atrophy or shrinkage of tissues. Such shrinkage overlaps considerably with the atrophy that occurs in normal aging and thus cannot be used for an individual patient to make a diagnosis of AD. Although attempts are under way to develop blood and cerebral spinal fluid (CSF) tests to diagnose AD, the clinician today can honestly say to the patient and family only that, having eliminated other possible causes, the diagnosis is probable AD. Using modern criteria, clinicians experienced in diagnosing patients with AD are correct approximately 85 percent of the time when their clinical diagnoses of probable AD are confirmed by tissues examined after death.

ALZHEIMER'S DISEASE

In 1907, Alois Alzheimer described the first case of AD, which he called a "peculiar disease of the cerebral cortex" (Alzheimer, 1907). This paper attracted attention because it described a woman who was 51 years old, and, although senile dementia in older individuals had been recognized for some time, the occurrence of a similar syndrome in a younger individual was unusual. Moreover, Alzheimer described not only the clinical course but also the pathological changes in the brain, which included loss of nerve cells in association with what we now call senile plaques and neurofibrillary tangles. We still diagnose AD by examination of brain tissue using the same cell stains and looking for the same pathological features that Alzheimer used more than eighty years ago. The chance of suffering from AD increases dramatically as one ages. Estimates of the number of people suffering from Alzheimer's disease in this country alone reach as high as 4 million individuals (Office of Technology Assessment, 1987). The chance of suffering from Alzheimer's disease before the age of 65 is small, whereas the risk over the age of 85 may be as high as 50 percent (Evans et al., 1989).

CLINICAL FEATURES

Alzheimer's original patient first developed a change in personality characterized by increasing suspiciousness that continued on to frank paranoia as she became concerned about her physician's intentions about her well-being. Cognitive difficulties started with memory impairment but proceeded to involve language, including writing, reading, and speech. She died four and one-half years after the onset of the disease in a state in which she was unable to care for her own needs. Thus, the first reported patient with AD had both cognitive and noncognitive or behavioral symptoms. The major focus of clinical studies of AD has been the cognitive or neuropsychological impairments, although now attention is being paid to the behavioral or psychiatric dysfunction (Patterson et al., 1990).

COGNITIVE CHANGES

The most frequent initial symptom in AD is amnesia, most commonly the inability to remember recent events rather than remote events. Thus, the family rather than the patient will often complain that the patient has difficulty remembering names or faces, and performance at work or at home may be affected. Subtle changes in personality, and in "executive" or planning abilities, may appear early as well. Thus, patients may not be able to focus their attention or organize their lives as they were previously able to do.

As the disease progresses, other cognitive abilities are affected. The patient may have difficulties finding words and, eventually, may manifest frank aphasia—language impairment. The performance of skilled motor acts, such as cooking or driving, will be affected. In addition, visual and auditory perceptual difficulties may occur which may be particularly difficult for the clinician to detect but may be quite disabling. Although peripheral hearing and vision are not affected unless other disorders of ears or eyes exist, the patient may not be able to organize his or her perceptions of the world into a coherent model, and a complex scene may be distorted and seem simpler. As the disease progresses, these cognitive difficulties impair activities of daily living. First, complex, or instrumental, activities like shopping, managing financial affairs, and work will be affected, and eventually, basic activities such as bathing, toileting, and feeding. In the end stages, the patient may not recognize any caregivers, including spouses he or she may have known for half a century. Finally, affected individuals may become incontinent and unable to feed themselves, becoming completely dependent on others.

BEHAVIORAL FEATURES

Subtle changes in personality, such as suspiciousness or irritability, may be the first signs of AD. As the disease progresses, depression or other affective symptoms may become prominent. Later in the disease, frank psychosis with hallucinations (usually visual) and delusions may occur. The hallucinations may be frightening or may be accepted by the patient as natural, such as the presence of children in the room.

The delusions frequently center around the loss of objects (e.g., the patient believes that people are stealing things) and, unfortunately, are often directed at the caregiver. In some patients, behavioral management may not be adequate and psychotropic drugs can be used, although with these drugs the clinician will often walk a thin line between therapeutic benefit and toxicity, including the possibility of further impairing the patient's cognitive abilities.

BIOLOGICAL FEATURES

The inventory of nerve cell populations affected by the disorder has grown since Alzheimer's original descriptions of pathology in the cerebral cortex of his patient's brain. Moreover, our understanding of the molecular biology of the intra- and extracellular changes has increased dramatically.

We know now that neural dysfunction and eventual cell death occur in several brain regions that are likely important for producing the cognitive and psychiatric aspects of the disease. In addition to the neocortex, these other areas of the brain include the hippocampus, amygdala, basal forebrain, locus coeruleus, and raphe nuclei. The pathology in the cortex is known to focus on temporoparietal areas, which may explain the language and visuospatial difficulties from which the patients suffer (Cummings and Benson, 1983; Price et al., 1986).

In several brain regions, we know which neurotransmitters are associated with the dying neurons—for example, acetylcholine in the base of the brain. One of the main changes in an Alzheimer's diseased brain is the presence of senile plaque, which is known to be composed of a core made of amyloid, surrounded by nerve cell processes and, finally, glial cells. The amyloid is composed primarily of a 42–amino-acid protein that itself is the breakdown product of a larger amyloid precursor protein. A gene on chromosome 21 produces this normal cellular protein. The neurofibrillary tangles are intracellular structures composed of several proteins, including tau. The consequence of the presence of plaques and tangles on cell health are not really understood, and we still do not understand why nerve cells die, the key biological question in AD.

Our knowledge of what causes AD is not adequate enough to be helpful in developing therapeutic interventions. Since shortly after Alzheimer described his first case, we have known that genes contribute to the disease in some families. Today we know that there are probably several different genetic forms of AD. In one form, the gene causing Alzheimer's disease has been located, using a process called "linkage analysis" to chromosome 21. The relationships between the amyloid precursor protein and the gene that causes AD on chromosome 21 are not understood. In some cases, the gene causing the disorder may be an abnormality in amyloid precursor protein gene (Goate et al., 1991), and in others, different genes on the 21st or other chromosomes may produce the disease which just happen to be on the same chromosome. Although not all families have a well-defined genetic risk, understanding the genetic mechanisms in the rare families with a clear-cut autosomal dominant form will help us to understand the pathogenesis of all AD.

The second major clue that we have to understanding the etiology of AD is its relationship to normal aging. As mentioned above, older individuals have a greater risk for developing the disease. As we all age, neurons die and we develop some plaques and tangles. The complex relationship between normal aging in the brain and Alzheimer's disease remains to be elucidated.

Epidemiology has provided certain clues to etiology, although we do not yet know whether these clues are genuine or are misleading artifacts of study design. Previous head injuries may predispose to AD. In some epidemiological studies, people who smoke have less chance of getting AD. No clear-cut evidence for a role for environmental toxins has been found in AD, although speculations concerning a role for exposure to aluminum continue. Other theories relate the cause of Alzheimer's disease to a novel infectious particle or disturbance in the immunological system. These ideas are scientifically heuristic, but they are too speculative to affect clinical practice today.

RESEARCH ISSUES FOR THE FUTURE

BIOLOGICAL RESEARCH

The critical biological research questions are: What causes AD, and why do nerve cells die? The presence of plaques and tangles provides clues to explore, although we do not yet know whether these are primarily related to the disease process or are epiphenomena. Genetic studies are likely to provide key information about this process of cell death. These studies should also allow us to offer counsel to family members of affected patients on their risks of developing the disease. Currently, in the autosomal dominant form, individuals have a 50 percent risk of developing AD. Additional linkage studies may lead us to the development of tests that allow us to inform asymptomatic individuals that their risks are actually much greater, close to 100 percent—or much less, close to 0 percent—as has been done in Huntington's disease. The identification in individual families of a specific genetic abnormality should make it possible to inform an individual, with almost complete accuracy, whether or not he or she has the disease gene.

Next, we need to understand not just *why* nerve cells die, but also *which* nerve cells die. At this level of analysis, understanding the characteristics of the specific cell populations that die is key to developing drug therapies. For example, neurotransmitters are the chemical basis for cell communication that underlies our thought processes. Replacing missing neurotransmitters with drugs may improve neural function, and enhancing mechanisms for maintaining cell viability may slow progression of the disease. Certain cell populations require specific growth factors to remain viable. The chemical messenger of these basal forebrain cells includes acetylcholine, a neurotransmitter that we know (from animal studies) is important for memory. Drugs to enhance cholinergic function are currently being developed. For example, nerve growth factor was first identified in the 1960s and was later identified as important for the health of cells in the basal forebrain. Therapeutic attempts using nerve growth factor are already under way to enhance the viability of these cells that die in AD. Thus, the characterization of the affected cells will allow the development of more effective therapies.

CLINICAL RESEARCH

Probably the most important clinical research question is whether AD is a single disease or multiple disorders. The genetic information we have gained suggests tht there is, in fact, heterogeneity. Physicians are aware that the use of an eponym, like Alzheimer's, to describe an illness usually reflects inadequate knowledge about classification. Thus, before we embark on finding diagnostic tests and therapies, we need to keep an open mind about whether we are seeking the treatment of a single entity or whether there may be multiple different entities with different therapies waiting to be discovered.

After answering questions that facilitate classification of diseases, major goals for clinical researchers are obviously the development of more effective diagnostic tests and therapies. Already under way are efforts to develop a specific diagnostic test for AD by examining cerebrospinal fluid and blood. Moreover, functional brain imaging, such as SPECT (single photon emission computerized tomography), and PET (positron emission tomography), which allows us to watch the brain at work in life, is the subject of intense and expensive research. Patterns of temporoparietal cortical dysfunction visible in life correspond to the distribution of pathology in death. As yet, however, none of these tests has led to a more specific clinically useful diagnostic test.

Basic biological studies are leading to clinical trials of agents that may prove to be of benefit to patients with AD. Currently we have no approved medications using modern standards of efficacy that significantly influence the progress of the disease. Tacrine, a drug that may enhance the function of acetylcholine by blocking its breakdown, has been rejected by the Food and Drug Administration as inappropriate for clinical use because the risks of using it appear to outweigh the possible benefits. Nevertheless, in the years to come we will likely be seeing medications that do provide some symptomatic relief. And the hope for the future is to develop therapies that actually slow the progression of disease.

HEALTH SERVICES RESEARCH

Although biological research for the future promises interventions that may influence the course of the disease, we do not yet know if and when they will develop. Thus, it is exceedingly important that we examine critically the manner in which we currently care for victims of the disease and their families.

There is no disease that better illustrates the fragility of our current health care system than AD. A system that focuses on intensive care and cure, rather than chronic care and management, is ill designed to deal with dementia. The challenges of finding a balance between inpatient hospital, community, and institutional long-term care must be addressed by research that assesses the impact of interventions on the quality of lives of patients and their families.

A spirit of innovation is alive in communities, resulting in programs such as dementia-specific day care programs and nursing home special-care dementia units in institutions. Access to such innovative programs is often limited, however, by a lack of information available to caregivers to help them select programs to meet their needs.

CONCLUSION

Dementia is a challenge for patients, families, professionals, and society. The very characteristics of dementia as a medical syndrome—such as its frequency, occurrence in old age, genetic nature, effects on competence, and progressive and often irreversible nature—generate profound ethical and public policy issues. In framing ethical and public policy debates regarding dementia, however, it is important to balance the professional's perspective of the illness with the individual patient's and family's experience with suffering from one's dementia, a subject addressed in the next two chapters.

REFERENCES

Alzheimer, A. (1907). Uber eine eigenartige Erkrandung der Hirnrinde. *Allgemeine Zeitschrift für Psychiatrie und PsychischiGerichtliche Medizin, 64*:146–148.

Cummings, J.L., and Benson, D.F. (1983). *Dementia: A Clinical Approach*. Boston: Butterworths.

Evans, D.A., Funkenstein, H.H., Albert, M.S., Scherr, P.A., Cook, N.R., Chown, M.J., Hebert, L.E., Hennekens, C.H., and Taylor, J.O. (1989). Prevalence of Alzheimer's disease in a community population of older persons. *Journal of the American Medical Association, 262*:2551–2556.

Goate, A., Chartier-Harlin, M.-C., Mullan, M., Brown, J., Crawford, F., Fidani, L., Giuffra, L., Haynes, A., Irving, N., James, L., Mant, R., Newton, P., Rooke, K., Roques, P., Talbot, C., Pericak-Vance, M., Roses, A., Williamson, R., Rossor, M., Owen, M., and Hardy, J. (1991). Segregation of a missense mutation in the amyloid precursor protein gene with familial Alzheimer's disease. *Nature, 349*:704–706.

Office of Technology Assessment, Congress of the United States (1987). *Losing a Million Minds: Confronting the Tragedy of Alzheimer's Disease and Other Dementias*. Washington, D.C.: U.S. Government Printing Office.

Patterson, M.B., Schnell, A., Martin, R.J., Mendez, M.F., Smyth, K.A., and Whitehouse, P.J. (1990). Assessment of behavioral and affective symptoms in Alzheimer's disease. *Journal of Geriatric Psychiatry and Neurology, 3*:21–30.

Price, D.L., Whitehouse, P.J., and Struble, R.G. (1986). Cellular pathology in Alzheimer's and Parkinson's disease. *Trends in Neuroscience, 9*:29–33.

3

THE EXPERIENCE OF BEING DEMENTED

Joseph M. Foley

What do demented people experience? What does their condition mean to them? What is their reaction to it? What are their gratifications? What are their frustrations? Does dementia allow the development of coping strategies available to other people with afflictions? These are urgent questions without satisfactory answers at present.

There still persists in some quarters the unfortunate misperception that the demented person is unaware of the fact of dementia. Anyone who spends any time at all with demented people, especially those who are less than severely demented, knows that at least some patients are aware that they are in intellectual decline, that they have a disease that is progressive, that their behavior is abnormal, and that other people are being affected by their condition. Such relatively full awareness, although demonstrable more easily in the early or middle stages, can persist into the later or more severe stages. In contrast to such patients, some patients have no awareness at all that anything is wrong. Some become hostile when challenged, but others try to be reasonable and respond kindly to the concerns of the families and the professionals. They seem to have a true, probably neurologically based anosognosia, an inability to recognize or acknowledge their dementia.

In between these poles are infinite variations. Some patients, aware that something is wrong, refuse to admit it and resort to denial and concealment, a pattern not unfamiliar in other kinds of human disease. As Henig (1988) noted:

As the disease progresses, and patients become more and more incapable of thinking in abstract terms, remembering, or expressing themselves, they may continue to develop tricks to avoid placing themselves in revealing situations. If asked a direct question ["How old are you Mrs. Collins?"] they deflect a direct answer that might give away their ignorance ["How old do you think I am?". . .]. . . . Other patients with Alzheimer's disease invent elaborate answers bearing little relation to reality or to the original question—a trick psychiatrists call "confabulation." . . . Some patients may deny that anything is wrong with their memory or ability to think. And some patients may engage in another defensive trick called "perseveration."

An individual who perseverates . . . returns over and over again during an interview to the first answer, the first story, the first word that had been right or nearly right, and tries to stick with it in hopes of it being right again. (pp. 136–137)

Some patients are aware only part of the time. Some are aware that all is not right, but cannot comprehend the nature of the problem or its significance for themselves or others. There is a full spectrum of emotional response (see Sacks, 1990). Some are placid and seemingly resigned; others are agitated and angry. Here, also, there are variations in content and intensity at different times. Placidity may prevail for hours or days or even weeks, to be succeeded by agitation. Some patients, seemingly completely uncommunicative and badly demented, may open windows of clarity for minutes or hours.

When we make efforts to help a patient or a patient's family, it is important that we know the nature and intensity of the cognitive deficits, but it is equally, if not more important that we know what the patient is thinking and feeling. The temptation to categorize such experiences with preconceptions is to be resisted. They must be explored in depth with each patient.

CASE PRESENTATION

F.G., a 72-year-old widower, has had Alzheimer's disease for five years. As will be clear in the excerpts from an interview, presented below, he is articulate and willing to serve as a teaching and research subject. No more than any one person can, he illustrates all the subjective experiences of the demented patient; but he exemplifies the kind of information available to the professional who thinks it important enough to pursue.

The patient is a university graduate, expert in the field of telecommunications, a contributor to the literature of his field. He is on good terms and in frequent contact with his four grown children, all of whom live in other parts of the country. He referred himself to our ElderHealth Center at age 68 because he was troubled by memory problems.

Previously very good at people's names, he found himself groping for the names even of people he knew very well. He had missed some appointments, to his great embarrassment. Only later did we learn from his secretary and his accountant, whom we interviewed with his permission, that the quality of his financial skills had declined over a year's period. He had tried to make some peculiar investments, had moved his money around inappropriately, and had misplaced checks and negotiable securities. This was in sharp contrast to his previous meticulous concern with business affairs. Yet in the preceding few months he had published in professional journals.

He lived alone in an apartment, swam and bicycled daily, visited his office several times a week, skied the Rockies in the winter, played the carillon at his church, attended symphony concerts and art exhibits. He drove his own car, and only a few months before this interview had made an automobile round trip of 1,600 miles.

On examination, except for mild hypertension, he had no physical abnormalities. He was pleasant, friendly, rather intense but appropriate. Language was generally very fluent, but infrequently he held up in the middle of a sentence and seemed perplexed, losing track of what he was to say. As the interview continued, this became more prominent, and in the succeeding years he continued to be very vulnerable to fatigue. He could comprehend what was said to him, used words correctly, had a spotty performance on the Boston Naming test, read and wrote without difficulty. He was oriented for person and place, was hesitant but accurate for time, was able to carry out purposeful movements, and reacted to stimuli. Proverb interpretation and abstractions were done less well than expected. Calculations were unimpaired, even for long division, but he had trouble with the 100-7 test when he got down to 58. He could remember only one of three objects after an intervening task, and could remember six numbers forward and three backward. When he failed a task, he begged to try it again, and sometimes succeeded the second time.

The "dementia work-up" was initiated, but the results showed no evidence of a reversible or arrestable process. A discussion was held; he heard our opinion that this was Alzheimer's disease, listened to our explanation, and asked for further literature on the subject. We mapped out a plan of action, with which he concurred.

Over the next four and one-half years he remained relatively stable, except for increasing problems with language, memory, and judgment. After some awkward financial problems, he agreed to relinquish the financial details but not overall control to his accountant and lawyer. After some slight bother with his automobile on a trip, he agreed to drive only locally except when a close friend or relative accompanied him. Yet he continued to live alone, have weekly cordial dinners with his divorced wife (who died shortly before the videotape was made), swam and bicycled daily, continued to play the carillon and to attend concerts and exhibitions. He volunteered to be a research subject for the study of Alzheimer's disease and was actively interested in new information about the disease.

In the week before the interview presented below, he went to a convention of carillonneurs on the East Coast. He had arrived in Cleveland by Amtrak early in the morning of the day of the interview. In the course of the trip he was unable to remember the name "Amtrak," the name of the train station, or the part of the city in which it was located. He walked four miles in the general direction of downtown, ultimately found the station, and arranged sleeping accommodations for the trip home. He was able to tell about this part of the experience but could not be specific about details.

Some of the more instructive parts of the interview follow:

JMF: Frank, you've been coming in to see me now for the last few years. Could you tell us your perception of why it is that you come to visit me, why you come to the Center: What is your perception of what it is that is troubling you?

FG: My perception is that the Center is very much wide awake on the various diseases that affect people in my situation and I have respected that and I find it very helpful to be told by you and your people what it is that I'm having.

JMF: What is your own idea of the trouble you have? Could you verbalize for us what you believe your trouble to be?

FG: Well, my touble is Alzheimer's disease because (chuckle) you people have told me that. Well, that's the name of it and the trouble I have is an occasional loss of memory and I otherwise really don't have a problem.

JMF: You've had the memory problem, then. Can you give us any examples of where your memory trouble bothers you or how it bothers you?

FG: Well I think anybody who has lots of friends and sometimes forgets the friends' names or has medical assistance and forgets the name of the doctor that may be working on him has [sic] very annoying. Now, it hasn't happened for quite a while now.

JMF: Do you get into more than embarrassment with it? Does it ever cause you inconvenience? Do you miss any appointments? Have you lost out on any engagements you might have had?

FG: I would say occasionally but there has been no instance of that in the last couple of years.

JMF: How about your friends and associates? Are they aware that you have any problem at all? I know your immediate family does.

FG: My immediate family does. Some of the people that I enjoy being with I have acquainted with the fact that this may happen. But it hasn't happened lately.

JMF: What do you tell them? Your friends . . .

FG: I tell them straight off that it's a disease, it's noncurable from what I've learned from you. I have it, it's not contagious. I'm doing real fine and I'm going to work hard for what life I have still.

JMF: What limitations does this thing put upon you? Do you feel any limitations because of your awareness of having the trouble?

FG: I would say no because the trouble has not advanced to a point where I would feel bad about driving my car. I've checked my driving and it's normal. People I know some know of this condition. Some do not. I don't spread it around because in normal ways there's no indication of something being abnormal. Right at this moment it's not a problem.

JMF: What about your financial affairs? Who handles them for you?

FG: Well, I handle my own financial affairs. I have a secretary who picked me up this morning at the train. She does the study work and I sign the papers. I'm in charge.

JMF: You remember that we all met together a few months ago, your secretary, you and I—and we agreed that certain documents that had been going to you were instead to be mailed to your secretary's office. Do you remember that?

FG: I now remember it, now that your remind me.

JMF: You used to do a good deal of writing.

FG: Yes. I've been published in a number of ways including a couple books that I got (long pause) in . . .

JMF: What were they about?

FG: Well, they were about my knowledge . . . I don't know exactly how to explain this but . . . it was how to . . . make or . . . your knowledge of the art . . . do well for a company that needed that sort of thing into application . . . and . . . It's fairly complicated, that's why I'm stuttering around about it. I'm no longer doing that. It's gone way beyond me, the things that are being done in that . . . that . . . telecommunications is what we call it.

JMF: May I ask you about your memory at this moment?

At this point in the interview, he was asked about orientation. He could give the month, the day of the month, the day of the week. When asked the year he replied:

FG: That's a good question. Ah . . . 90 ah . . . (laugh). I should put that right off my head.

JMF: There are times when I've talked to you in the past few months, times when you can give me that information right away, with no hesitation and great accuracy and other times when you seem to have a lot of difficulty giving it. Are you aware of this, that there are times when you do very well and times when you fumble and stutter?

FG: Of course. I don't like to fumble.

JMF: What does it feel like when you have to fumble?

FG: Well, it's embarrassing if you're trying to fumble with somebody else around or I mean if you fumble automatically. It's also unfortunate for the person with the problem to recognize it and if you can diagnose what you can do to get out of the problem at that moment, you do it. And if you don't, you're unhappy.

JMF: You mean there are tricks you can use to get yourself through it?

FG: I don't look at it that way, but I get myself out of that situation.

JMF: I didn't mean that in any pejorative way.

FG: Oh no. I understand.

JMF: We'll put it in a professional term and ask are there stratagems for avoiding it.

FG: Well, the stratagems. I think I've discovered some of those but I can't tell you what they are. Not that I don't want to, but I've been able as a single person with Alzheimer's disease to handle that all right so far. Now I recognize that this may get worse but on a whole week of traveling and quite interesting things where I had to take participation I had no problems whatsoever and enjoyed it with my colleagues.

JMF: Is there anything that makes it easier for you to handle this problem of yours?

FG: I think the thing that I do and what others possibly also do is to make notes of the things that look as if they're not being handled properly and I . . . Other than that, I really don't have a problem at this point in time with people and recognizing names. That seems to be flowing along OK, so . . .

JMF: Can I quiz you about that just a bit?

FG: Sure.

JMF: Can you tell me who is the President of the United States?

FG: Oh, Lord! Thinking about George. Well I just read it this morning but it's gone.

JMF: Would his name be Bush?

FG: (Big laugh) Absolutely. I should have had it in the first place but . . .

JMF: Who is the Vice President? What's his name?

FG: The Vice President. Let's see. I can't do that off hand and (long pause). Now what was your question again?

JMF: What things help you handle this difficulty that you have? The memory trouble, the awareness of the disease and so forth? What things in your life make it easier to deal with?

FG: I think understanding people. When your closest friends have not been put in a position where they don't know about it. I'd rather have them know, know if there is a problem. Now the good thing is that at this point there's been no difficulty that I have to worry about. I mean I'm driving my car and my bike. I'm swimming. I'm doing the things that I want to do. I still belong to the church and I still go to the Cleveland Orchestra concerts and there's no driving problem.

JMF: What makes it hard for you? Are there any things that make it difficult for you to put up with this problem of yours?

FG: Well, the difficult thing is that it has a tail end to Alzheimer's and I'm not too anxious to get to that point. I'm glad to know what I have. I don't know any particular cure for this that I've been told about. There's no medicine that I know about. I think the fact that you know you have a disease that's going to knock you off your stool sometime is a depressing matter.

JMF: Do you get depressed?

FG: Not particularly because I'm normally happy about what I'm doing.

JMF: Do you think about it very much?

FG: No, because there it is. Why think about it?

The patient is able, despite the circumlocutions, awkward phrasing, and non sequiturs, to tell us a great deal. (1) He knows something is wrong with him. (2) He accepts that it is Alzheimer's disease because he has been so informed by people he trusts. He knows it is incurable and he is concerned about the end result. (3) He has elected to live his life, do the best he can, and get gratification of the sort he enjoys. (4) He has some understanding of what helps him and what hurts him in his determination to cope with his affliction. (5) He is aware of some, but not all, of his deficiencies. He fails to remember (actively denies?) many of his failures. Although he makes the statement several times that "there are no problems now," he accepts that he has had problems when they are called to his attention.

This patient is not the typical patient with progressive dementia, but we may reasonably ask if there is any such typical patient. There is reason to believe that each patient, if we are able to delve deep enough and long enough, will have an individuality that will elude any of our efforts to find the "typical." Our patient, F.G., is exceptional in many ways. He is coping very well; many patients do not cope as well as he does, whether because of the nature of the brain involvement, or because of medical or social complications, or because they did not carry into their dementia the kind of resources that are uniquely his. He is sufficiently articulate and able to carry on a conversation to give us some idea of the feelings and insights he has about his dementia.

I submit that if we are going to talk about ethics in relation to dementia, we must know not just about cognitive capacity but also about awareness, feelings, and emotional reactions to the personal and social consequences of dementia. I fear that sometimes we assume too much. We too often assume that the absence of emotional display means that no emotion is being experienced. We too often assume that because communication is absent, internal mental process has stopped. This is an area worthy of further extended systematic study, especially because it is crucial to any considerations of rights or obligations, and of the morality of decisions involving demented people.

I would like to move toward, without every arriving at, answers to the following questions. What awareness do demented patients have of their deficiencies? What emotional responses to they have to their deficiencies? What is the relationship between insight and emotional response? What is the relevance of insight or lack thereof to the rights and obligations of demented patients?

The literature on the subject is remarkably scarce. Insight is the capacity to discern the true nature of the situation or, as applied to dementia, the recognition of the fact, degree, and implications of one's own illness. Insight as a phenomenon in the neuroses and psychoses has been discussed extensively, virtually ad infinitum. In dementia, only passing reference can be found. I have been unable to locate any systematic treatment of the issue in the literature of geriatrics, psychology, or gerontological psychiatry. This is remarkable because so much of the management of the demented patient depends on his or her capacity to understand what is wrong.

The most notoriously difficult patients to manage are those who believe there is nothing wrong with them and then act, often destructively, on that erroneous presumption. Such patients can be even more troublesome than those who are aware of a deficiency but actively deny it, explaining away their behavior by rationalizations, subterfuges, or downright lies. I suspect that part of the reason for the paucity of information about insight is that the issue does not lend itself to quantification by instruments of the sort so beloved by the physicians, nurses, psychologists, and social scientists who work in the field of dementia. To my knowledge, there is no insight scale, or inventory, or status-generating numbers to give maximum consolation and minimum real information to the testers. Information about insight must be gained by history, by repeated observation, and by sometimes painful discussion with the patient.

In understanding many human conditions we have been helped by the storyteller or the artist. I think of these accounts or portrayals as a kind of modeling of reality. Much in the manner of mathematical or computer models, we seek to formulate hypotheses for an understanding of reality. Lear on the moor is a splendid model of delirium, precipitated by multiple personal and climatic stressors. Yeats described transient global amnesia in Father Gilligan. Sometimes literature and art get closer to the reality of human behavior than do testing instruments that are of necessity arbitrary and impersonal, however desirable they may be for purposes of classification and research.

A remarkable book published in Dutch in 1984 came to the attention of American readers when an English translation appeared in this country in 1988. A work of fiction by the Dutch writer Bernlef (1988), it is a first-person account of Maarten, a 71-year-old Dutchman living with his wife in Gloucester, Massachusetts.

It starts from his first hazy awareness that something is wrong with him. It tells of the perplexity, cover-ups, rationalizations, justifications, and distortions as he tries to deal with his new state of mind, with the inconsistencies of his daily life, and with the reactions of people around him, especially his wife.

He is a good man; he does not try deliberately to deceive, and only in delusional panic does he strike out. He is intermittently aware of the irrationality of his behavior, and he struggles to understand, but with a failing mind that defeats his efforts. He waits by the window for the children to pass on their way to school, becomes alarmed when they fail to appear, and, having to be told it is Sunday, wonders why that possibility had not occurred to him. He awakens at night, can't get back to sleep, gets up to read, and then can't explain to his wife why he is fully dressed instead of in his dressing gown.

Years after he has retired he puts material in his briefcase and goes off to work, winding up at a deserted house waiting impatiently and indignantly for his colleagues to appear. He reflects, "It worries me that you can suddenly be so cut off from the most ordinary everyday actions" (p. 17). Another: "I can think of nothing but vanished memories, and therefore dare not think of the past any more. . . . Perhaps it is only temporary, perhaps they will come back. Memories can sometimes be temporarily inaccessible, like words, but surely they can never disappear completely during your lifetime? But what are they exactly, memories? They are a bit like dreams. You can retell them afterwards but what they really are, whether they are real, you don't know, no one does" (p. 19).

On another occasion, he is struggling to find a word of explanation: "Denial. Of course! Another word for refusal. Six letters beginning with d. I've been chewing on that for a whole hour. It is as if the winter air is widening my veins. Maybe that's what it is, hardening of the arteries. You become forgetful. It's part of old age. . . . More a general feeling of unease than a specific symptom. But no, it would be nonsense to think that there is something really wrong. 'I'm still going strong!' . . . I must not make a habit of this, of talking out loud to myself" (p. 25).

His wife tells a friend: " 'I'm really worried. You can't see there's anything wrong with him. But that makes it all the more alarming. Sometimes he tells me things about us that I was never a part of. As if I were a different person in his eyes. And then suddenly he can't remember a whole chunk of his own past. I feel so helpless because I don't know how to help him' " (p. 33).

His wife, again, asks how he feels. " 'Like a ship,' I say, 'a ship, a sailing vessel that is becalmed. And then suddenly there is a breeze. I am sailing again. Then the world has a hold on me again and I can move along with it.' " His wife replies, " 'I find it so hard to imagine, Maarten. I can't see anything wrong with you at all. It is if you were looking at something, at something that I can't see. Are you afraid of those moments? What exactly happens to you then?' " He says, " 'I don't know. I can't remember. Only that feeling of a sudden heaviness, as if I am sinking through everything and there is nothing to hold on to' " (p. 64).

" *'We're going for a walk, Robert,'* " Maarten says to his dog. His wife says, " 'Marten, the doctor says you're not to go out.' " He replies, " 'Since when does a doctor decide whether I go or do not go? I'm not sick. At least I don't feel sick.' " She warns, " 'You're a little confused. You might get lost.' " " 'Get lost?,' " he says. " 'Yes, because you sometimes forget which way to go.' " He says, " 'Not when Robert is there. He knows the way home no matter where he is, even from the center of Boston.' " His wife responds, " 'The other day you lost Robert when you were out.' " He reflects, "Clearly she is inventing stories to test me. If I confirmed them I would be lost. I would lose myself in her fabrications. Maybe that doctor of hers told her to do it. Try to find out if he can still distinguish reality from fiction. A test. Better not reply. Better not respond to anything" (p. 69).

As his mind disintegrates, Maarten still verbalizes the disorder of his thinking and feeling self—the misinterpretation of the actions of others, the frustrations of his own failures, the hallucinations, the delusions, the loss of the significance of places, the failure of sequences in time, the confusion about who other people really are.

Do demented people think and feel this way? We have no way of knowing for sure, but we can think of this as a kind of model. It makes comprehensible the behavior of this particular demented person and gives us a possible understanding of what manner of thoughts demented people have and how they see and react to the world and the people about them. I emphasize that this remarkable story tells of only one demented person. This is only his unique clouded insight.

Clinical experience is never as deep as fiction, but it may be as dramatic. The very nature of dementia makes it difficult and in some cases impossible to learn what thought processes and what feelings lie behind the distorted behaviors. Dementia is in essence a decline from a previously attained intellectual level.

There are all grades of severity of intellectual loss, disturbance, and affect. Afflicted patients will respond in many different ways to the stressors of the environment. Yet we can make some generalizations about what the demented person thinks and feels.

1. Some patients have a full awareness that something is wrong with their intellectual capacities and preserve an awareness to some degree through the course of their disease. A physician of 62, a friend of mine, came into my office, sat down, and calmly said, "I have Alzheimer's disease." She had slow progression of intellectual failure over a period of four to five years during which she continued to see some patients. She lived alone, drove a car, and attended social gatherings. Then her distintegration progressed more rapidly; but even when she was suffering from severe language disorder, she would mutter "Damn Alzheimer's." Following her death, nine years after her earliest symptoms, autopsy showed Alzheimer's disease.

2. Some patients have no awareness of any deficiency in their intellectual state and act accordingly even as they disintegrate. A 63-year-old married woman, with classical manifestations, listened to accounts of her disordered functions and explanations of her disease process, went to the library to read about it, agreed that the concerned professionals were sincere and confident, but declared that she herself saw nothing wrong at all. She acted on this delusion of normalcy, and as the disease progressed, all her actions were consistent with the conviction that she was normal. Not surprisingly, she resorted to delusional and paranoid thinking, feeling, and behavior, and it became necessary to supervise and control her. Five years after the onset of her symptoms, she said to me at the beginning of the office visit, with a charming smile and appropriate gesture, "I don't know what I'm doing here but there's no sense fighting about it. He'd bring me anyhow (pointing to her husband)." Her recount of her present daily activities was as they were ten years ago, with some transposition of places and some intergenerational confusion. She was totally uninfluenced by an effort to get her back to reality. She talked vaguely of a conspiracy between me

and her husband to have her certified as crazy. She was, in fact, clearly psychotic.

3. Some patients, aware that something is wrong, actively deny it and set up schemes of rather transparent concealment, convincing themselves that they are successful. A 62-year-old salesman got his wife to come on selling trips, and he represented her behind-the-scenes work as his own. Unable to cite the formerly well-known prices, he invented excuses for going out to talk to his wife about them. As the disease worsened, he then naively tried to deceive her.

4. The above examples of awareness, nonawareness, and denial are exceptional in the purity of their content and in their persistence. The far more common clinical example is far less pure and much more subject to variations through the course of the illness and the stressors that accompany it. A very familiar problem is the patient who has good insight at the beginning and then loses it, to end in either non-awareness or denial or both. Recognition of one's own cognitive failure often produces anxiety or depression, which can immobilize or distort coping mechanisms and produce superimposed decline in function, reversible if identified for what it truly is. Another familiar problem is the patient whose affective responses are blunted from the very beginning, who may or may not know but who cares little or not at all. Such patients are frequently passive and cooperative, even at a time when only small intellectual damage has been done, and they are frequently able to carry on a reasonable conversation with good understanding.

But most people are a mixture, and the variations from time to time are very great. We have often heard a family member say, in awe and embarrassment about the behavior of a new elderly patient at the first visit to the center, "I don't believe it, doctor. We haven't seen him this good for a whole year." The patient has risen to the occasion. The discrepancy between the history and the scores can be impressive in either direction. Variations in level of awareness, in affect, and in appropriateness of behavior involve a multitude of variants such as circadian rhythms, fatigue, fever, level of physical and social stimulation, biochemical and pharmacological changes of the internal environment, physical and social alterations of the external enviroment, and, of course, the severity of the disease process. Depending on the circumstances, the variation in intellectual and emotional fucntioning may occupy weeks, or days, or even hours or minutes. Some seemingly moderately advanced patients have windows of clarity which open and close irregularly and allow the normal personality and the normal intelligence to emerge from the shadow of the dementia.

In Alzheimer's disease, the most common of the progressive degenerative dementias, and some others, a language disorder almost inevitably occurs somewhere along the course, affecting production or comprehension or both. In some patients the language disorder is a herald of the dementia that may not arrive until months or even years later. Those not familiar with this effect—and they may be physicians, or worse (for the patient), the patient's spouse—will then impute the seeming nonsense of a conversation to intellectual decline. The language disorder may then represent another stressor, depending on its type, and result in frustration, isolation, anger, and depression, potentiating the cognitive deficits by inactivating the coping mechanism.

A 72-year-old with a relatively stable dementia was brought by her family because the condition had accelerated downward in recent weeks. There had been a subtle language disorder from the beginning, especially with naming people or things, and on examination it was clear that the process had worsened. In addition, crying episodes and brief shouting rages were occurring as communication became more difficult. Using familiar techniques of communication with dysphasic patients, we were able to determine that given enough time she could be made to understand more and we could interpret her production. We found that her husband had gone away for a week, as we had advised him to, and that her children had left her in the care of an attendant who fed and cleaned her, kept her dry, and accompanied her on her daily walks but spent most of the day ignoring her and watching television. The patient knew that there was a language disorder; not all victims of Alzheimer's disease have such awareness. Reeducation of the husband and family resulted in a gratifying reduction in the episodes of disordered behavior.

Those who concern themselves with ethical decisions for an individual person, or with the formulation of an ethical public or institutional policy for dementia, must have an awareness of the insights and feelings of demented patients as well as a knowledge of the cognitive defects. There must be recognition of the variability, from patient to patient, and from time to time in the same patient. It is important to identify functions that are lost, but even more so to identify functions that are preserved. Dementia per se does not always deny patients the right to participation in decisions about their own care, their own life, or their own health. In the formulation of public and institutional policy we must beware of simplifications and generalizations; we must recognize that individual demented persons have their own unique attributes and that, despite metaphors loosely thrown around, they each remain a person, with their own gratifications and frustrations, their own unique background, and their own unique destiny.

REFERENCES

Bernlef, J. (1988). *Out of Mind*, translated by Adrienne Dixon. Boston: David R. Godine.

Henig, R.M. (1988). *The Myth of Senility*. Glenview, Ill.: Scott, Foresman and Co.

Sacks, O. (1990). *The Man Who Mistook His Wife for a Hat*. New York: Harper Perennial.

4

SEEING
AND
KNOWING DEMENTIA

David H. Smith

I first met Martha when she was in her mid-50s: a lively and cultured New Yorker feeling out of context in the small midwestern university town to which she had moved with her husband, a professor. I met Martha when I was courting her daughter. Among my future wife's assets was her family setting.

Martha nursed her husband through a terminal illness, and within weeks of his death she moved back to New York. Trained as both a musician and a nurse, she soon began work at the New York Hospital and attended every concert, recital, or ballet performance she could. For six years I was in school in the area, so I shared in many of these outings during a season of blooming for us all. And the flowering continued through visits after my wife and I returned to live in the Midwest—through a sabbatical in Washington, the birth of grandchildren, and the ups and downs of lives.

Looking one's best mattered to Martha, as did high-quality performance. But she treasured "mute inglorious Miltons" and had little sympathy for public show that seemed to her to be without foundation. As a girl she had loved Rachmaninoff; one part of her soul was that of a romantic. In her 50s and 60s she was justifiably proud of her renewed ability to flourish in the metropolis.

In 1976 we spent a month in New Hampshire, and we joined Martha for a family reunion on the way home. We had not seen her for months; she seemed older and a little frail. At the big dining table her comments were not always on target. New York was no longer an unmixed bag of goodies, she said. We thought we should urge her to move to Indiana to be near us. At her Christmas visits during the following years, we pushed this option hard, for New York increasingly frightened her. Although she would not (or could not) bring herself to make the change, she agreed finally to the move on principle.

But before she could leave, in 1978, a woman from an apartment down the hall in New York called my brother-in-law. Her old friend Martha was behaving strangely, getting lost, forgetting where she was. Her son took her to a neurologist who did a brain scan that showed severe cerebral atrophy. But her daughter, sure her mother would respond to personal help, flew to be with her. Social graces remained: smiling at a visitor, laughing with the crowd, responding briefly and politely in conversation.

But at a reunion in her son's home, Martha remarked to her daughter, "Now, haven't I met you somewhere before?" Denial was no longer possible.

Should Martha stay with us? Our three children, then aged 6 to 11, filled the bedrooms, and it was clear Martha needed twenty-four-hour help. We had no financial reserve for an addition to the house or a move. What about a live-in companion in an apartment? We found an apartment, but the first companion was tough and unsympathetic, and her replacement, a student, could stay only a short time. Martha would go out and get lost; she would walk back and forth in the apartment, appearing purposeful but in reality doing nothing.

A more structured setting—physically controlled and with communal support—seemed essential, but good nursing homes were not easy to find. Most said they handled wanderers by restraining them in a chair. The thought of Martha tied down was agonizing. In a nearby town we found a lovely place that had Dutch doors on the rooms. Martha would start—and in fact she did start—outside the health care center of the facility, but within a week she was wandering outdoors wearing no coat on a winter's night. So she moved behind the door and the downward spiral continued: loss of concern with appearance, loss of control of body functions, loss of even a semblance of recognition of a loving daughter who drove to see her every week.

Two years later we went abroad on sabbatical. A seizure left Martha in a deep coma that might last for months. She died within hours of her daughter's departure from her bedside, but ten years later the hurt of her last years has not died.

This chapter reflects on and analyzes issues raised by the last two years of Martha's life. They are not the years she would choose to have remembered, or years that her family cherishes, but they are years in which we were in a crucible from which, perhaps, can come a usable alloy. I will organize my comments with reference to various moments or elements in the experience. Throughout, my main objective is to address the perspective from which we see dementia. For what we see determines who we are, what we hope for, and what we are able to do.

WHO COUNTS?

It is convenient to begin with a particularly hard issue: the question of identity, status, or ontology. How much do demented persons matter, and why do they matter? In a story in the *Washington Post*, a spouse remarked of her demented husband, "I took the pictures down of him with Hubert Humphrey and him with Lyndon Johnson and him with Jack Kennedy. This isn't the same person that was friends of people in high places and worked on programs with them" (Meyer, 1982a, p. A8). Similarly, I found myself wanting to say of Martha, "She's not the woman she once was"—meaning that observation rather literally. But, as always with literalism, the question of exactly what such a statement might mean calls for some brooding.

Probably everyone reading these pages realizes that there is at least one clear way of defining Martha's status, determining how much she counted after the dementia was well advanced. That method of reasoning proceeds roughly as follows: Personhood is a moral category. We properly and precisely call *persons* only those beings who are moral agents, able to take responsibility for their choices. Persons so denominated are of supreme moral value; indeed, they are the only certain value that we have.

Although I will distance myself from this way of reasoning in a moment, I want to note a couple of points in its favor. The first is clarity. The crisp moral concept of personhood helps us to answer the general question of who counts, and it gives us a clear starting point in discussing the demented. To be precise, it suggests that they are not persons, and they don't count. Even if we reject that view, offering a coherent rationale for rejection clarifies our options. Second, the choice of the human moral agent as the only certain value is hardly arbitrary. The logic behind it goes something like this: Our world of Jews, Christians, Hindus, Satanists, and Hedonists offers no agreement on any substantive external value such as God, justice, money, or sex. We can only agree on our right to disagree. But when I respect your right to disagree with me I am, in effect, agreeing to respect you as a person. Respect for persons, in short, seems to be the only shared value in a pluralistic society.

Finally, affirming that persons who are moral agents are the highest or trump value perhaps need not imply that they are the only value.

For example, H. Tristram Engelhardt, Jr., a brilliant exponent of person-centered morality, argues that persons "are persons . . . when they are self-conscious, rational, and in possession of a minimal moral sense" (Engelhardt, Jr., 1986, p. 109). Then he concedes the validity of a secondary "conferred" or "social" sense of personhood to cover valued beings who are not persons "in the strict sense" (pp. 115-123).

These points noted, I reiterate that if the person-focused view means anything at all, it means that at some point someone entering into a dementia begins to count less than, or have a different status than, the rest of us. Personhood hinges on the ability to accept responsibility. When that ability has disappeared—when it no longer makes sense to blame someone who is careless, inattentive, or out of touch—then there is no longer a person, and we should speak of a diminished form of moral, and perhaps legal, status. Thus a moral strategy originally designed for *inclusiveness* across divergent historical traditions and irreconcilable world views has a negative corollary: if you cannot be praised or blamed, you can't make quite the same moral claim on us that people we hold responsible can make.

If we apply this conceptual template to Martha, we might say that at some point she ceased to be a person; and that conclusion is correct given the stipulated understanding of what it means to be a person. She certainly ceased to be a moral agent. But what follows? That she need no longer be respected? That she was no longer part of the family? That it was incoherent to continue to love her? That she could make no reasonable claim on the resources or forbearances of the larger society? All these possible inferences seem to me to be self-evidently false, if not deeply immoral. Used as an engine of *exclusion*, the personhood theory easily leads to insensitivity, if not to great wickedness.

I claim that this personhood theory contradicts important moral sentiments aroused by dementia. That contradiction should push us to reexamine the premises on which the theory was founded, or at least the role it plays in normative ethics. I am saying, in effect, "OK, so she isn't a 'person,' so what?" If in response you try to specify claims that Martha no longer makes, I will challenge you on moral grounds independent of the personhood claim; if you can't specify any differences, then I wonder what significance the personhood criterion has. A restrictive, moral-agency–centered concept of personhood either does too much or too little. It is hard to use it in a discriminate way.

The core of the problem is that the personhood theory identifies human dignity too closely with individual moral agency. Thus it has trouble explaining the fundamental respect for dignity which parents owe to infants, which religious believers ascribe to God (and think God ascribes to them), or which we show to the demented. In these important contexts respect is rooted in the reality of relationship rather than in a property possessed by one of the parties. Dignity is foundational, and human dignity is distinctive, but its root is our engagements with one another, engagements that are often most deep when the issue is nurture or love rather than moral agency.

Thus I concede that Martha ceased to be a "person," but not that she lost her human dignity. Was she then the "woman she once was"? To answer that question, we must ask what gave her her identity, what made her what she was. The answer is that her identity arose in a series of relationships—with her parents, siblings, husband, children, and grandchildren. She was invested in those relations and dependent on them. And if those were the most obvious relations in Martha's life, they were complemented by involvements with nursing and music and dance, even with God. Her identity was constituted in those identifications and involvements, and it changed over time. The young mother in Paris in the 1930s was—and was not—the girl of twenty years earlier in Clearfield, Pennsylvania. In her decline, Martha changed again, so that at the end she was certainly not our ballet companion of fifteen years before. But she was still Martha, remaining identifiable as my wife's mother. Undignified as her life became, she retained human dignity.

I don't ask you to go through these reflections with me in order to minimize the change or loss in a victim of a progressive dementia. We became acutely aware of what the severely demented cannot do, or who they are not. Nor do I mean to imply that dementia is irrelevant to decisions about treatment, although exactly how and to what extent it may be relevant remains a vexed issue. At a minimum I would say that dementia may have the effect that some life-sustaining treatments can only be *perceived* as torture, and that perception is a formidable argument against using them. Appropriate forms of care are addressed elsewhere in this volume.

I do mean to say that because their dignity arises from their identifications and involvements, not solely from moral agency, the demented make full claims of justice as members of the human community. Although we should not treat them as if they were not demented, we also should not pretend that they are no longer part of our family or community.

THE IMPACT OF SUFFERING AND ISOLATION

If I am correct in my claim about the moral status of the demented, we have to face a second level of worry. Why is it that many thoughtful persons disagree with this analysis and commit themselves to a personhood theory? I think that part of the answer lies in a characteristic attitude toward suffering: If the demented are not persons, we can cease to identify with them and thus reduce our own suffering. The personhood theory as a belief system serves to insulate or protect us. Is that protection possible or desirable?

In fact, the story of dementia is the story of suffering. And this suffering is not brief and episodic; like all real suffering, it lasts. Dementia is not a brief, acute incident. It is essential to it to be stretched out in time and to seem endless. One spouse interviewed by the *Washington Post* years ago "talks about her life as though the active part of it is over. 'It isn't as if I have another, better life to look forward to. . . . Four years ago, I thought I did. But now I realize I don't.' " As another spouse puts it, "I can tell you that it is like a funeral that never ends" (Meyer, 1982b, p. A10).

I contend that the suffering involved in dementia is so severe because the demented experience isolation from others, loved ones, and self. The most visible aspect of this isolation which confronts any family is the complete absence of people to help out. That was our experience, and it recurs in the narratives of other family members. Writing in the *New York Times*, Phillip Boffey reported on a conference of families of Alzheimer's patients, convened by the National Institutes of Health, and summarized it by saying that these families complained about lack of skilled nursing facilities that accept and keep patients, the failure of government insurance to provide adequate coverage, and the absence of family counselors and support groups. "All too often (as they describe) the care provided is ignorant, indifferent, callous or even destructive" (Boffey, 1985, p. 15).

This isolation is not simply a matter of lack of practical help—as if that weren't enough. After his wife contracted Alzheimer's disease, Dr. Bernard Nathanson, a New York dentist, told a reporter, "The most devastating aspect of our lives has been the isolation. Nobody comes to visit us anymore, nobody calls, everybody ducks us. People are afraid" (Brozan, 1982, p. 1).

The patient is also isolated or separated from family members. One patient began to refuse to eat with his wife.

> He would say things to me like, "If you're going to be in here, I'm going in another room. I want a divorce. Who needs you?" See, he was feeling threatened, I suppose, and uneasy. I thought he was going through some kind of mid-life crisis or something. I was very unhappy about it, but I felt as if he were rejecting me. I find this a very common occurrence in talking to other women. They blame themselves. They think they have done something wrong. (Meyer, 1982b, p. A10)

Nothing makes this isolation clearer than nonrecognition, and the isolation readily becomes alienation, which easily turns to hostility. The spouse just quoted continues:

> I have been as many as seven people at one time to him. According to my function and the room I was in, he had me separated into all these different people. . . . He would warn me against the woman who had just given him a bath: "She's a bitch. Watch out for her. Watch out for the old lady who's out in the hall. She's always watching." He would warn me against me—the person he would perceive. He would warn me sometimes if I would kiss him, "Watch out! My wife may find out." (Meyer, 1982a, p. A8)

Finally, as the victims become more demented, they lose touch with past selves and identity. Perhaps the process reaches the point where it is merciful to forget, but the prolonged deterioration can be bewildering and terrifying. My wife's most painful memory of her mother's last days is of one of her last remarks. As they were seated at dinner, Martha leaned over and said, "You know, I think I am getting better." Martha *knew* that she was confused, that she was losing ground. Loss of control was as acutely painful within as without.

The best response to these forms of suffering is to find a way to offer reconciliation and community that will span the gap of estrangement and separation. In order to think in those terms, however, we must reject on moralistic and individualistic view of suffering which has been extraordinarily influential in medical ethics in the past fifty years. Who can forget Joseph Fletcher's account of the death of Jonathan Swift, written in 1954? It was, according to Fletcher, a

> horrible and degrading death. It was a death degrading to himself and to those close to him. His mind crumbled to pieces. It took him eight years to die while his brain rotted. He read the third chapter of Job on his birthday as long as he could see. "And Job spake, and said, Let the day perish when I was born, and the night in which it was said, There is a man child conceived." The pain in Swift's eye was so acute that it took five men to hold him down, to keep him from tearing out his eye with his own hands. For the last three years he sat and drooled. Knives had to be kept entirely out of his reach. When the end came, finally, his fits of convulsion lasted thirty-six hours. (Fletcher, 1954, pp. 174–175)

Of this history Fletcher commented, "Now, whatever may be the theological meaning of St. Paul's question, 'O death, where is thy sting?'

the moral meaning—in a word, the evil—of a death like that is only too plain" (p. 175).

Fletcher went on to celebrate moral personality as the core value in medical ethics, sounding a theme clearly recognizable in the more academic (and difficult) prose of Engelhardt forty years later. For these writers something must be done about suffering, and dementia with its destruction of the human moral agent becomes the greatest evil to be avoided. The *Post* series on Alzheimer's from which I have already quoted at length was graphic on this point. The stories quoted Dr. Robert Terry's observation that Alzheimer's disease is worse than cancer because, although cancer

> kills you, . . . it doesn't remove your very humanity, your intellect, your personality, your personal habits of hygiene. It doesn't turn you into a vegetable.
>
> It kills you, fine. We all have to face that. But I don't want to be destroyed as a human. It seems to me that that's the essence of why people were so ashamed for years of mental disease in general. Having cancer or tuberculosis was not sinful. But mental disease is—was. That's because it changes our very soul, our very spirit. It lessens our humanity.
>
> All diseases are depersonalizing to some extent. But you're still human. You can still respond to pain, anger, to hunger, to whatever and you're still thinking. But a person with a serious dementia is no longer human. He's a vegetable. That's devastating. Fearsome. Terrifying, to anyone who's ever seen it—the thought that that could happen to you. (Meyer, 1982b, p. A10)

Let me not pretend to be above these feelings; my own character is activistic, and the activism is morally, perhaps moralistically, charged. I want neither to be demented nor to discourage diagnostic and therapeutic innovation in the treatment of dementia. Still, when all is said and done, I find it hard to imagine that dementia will not continue as part of the human prospect. The fact of dementia is not to be erased.

The deeper problem with the moral-personality perspective is what it omits or fails to mandate. Because it sees moral personality as a value in a class by itself, it tends to think in dichotomous terms: either moral personality or nothing. Once the medical problem is posed in these moralistic terms, with the responsible in light and the demented in darkness, the door is open to practices and policies that are destructive to all—certainly to the untouchables. Our focus has shifted from helping demented persons to eradication of that absolute evil, dementia.

Ultimately the core of the mistake made by the moral-personality theorists is a misperception about what the world is like: They expect it to make moral sense. In particular, *suffering* must make moral sense, must be fitted into a morally coherent whole. Thus the suffering from dementia must fall into either of two categories. It may be *deserved*—in which case we have good moral grounds to shun patient and family. Or the suffering may be *pedagogical*—something we can learn from, a necessary obstacle for us to overcome on the way to maturity. Suffering makes moral sense in either of these theodicies. The trouble is that they are hard to swallow. While few victims of progressive dementia are saints, for even fewer is this a punishment that fits the crime. And dementia seems a particularly odd way to teach people to be moral (Smith, 1989).

In place of these perspectives an important strand of Western theism has insisted that the moral righteousness of the world is problematic. Job is tormented, and Christ ends up on the cross. From this point of view the appropriate response to suffering is trust in God and solidarity with other sufferers. The radical dichotomy is between God and humankind, not between the demented and the responsible. Compassion and loyalty to fellow sufferers become the chief moral requirements.

On these terms our moral perspective on dementia might more appropriately stress patience and community rather than frenetic attempts to get rid of the problem. Supposing dementia to be a core fact of life, we should be wondering how we can become the sorts of communities and selves which can cope with it. There is no denying a religious dimension to the question, at least in the West, for religious identity in the monotheistic traditions inevitably places the demented one in a larger social and temporal context. I can identify with you and myself in dementia precisely because my identity—and yours—lies in a relation to God rather than in the perfection of moral subjectivity. And I can have patience because trust in God makes sense.

Western theism may not be the only perspective that allows transcendence of moralistic activism. Indeed, many of the roots of the activist ethos are to be found in the Hebrew Bible and New Testament, in the Talmud and Augustine. But that older activism took place in the context of compassion, of shared conviction that as humans our lot is to suffer together. The older activism assumed that we should summon the courage to identify ourselves with the unfortunate. Because I am sympathetic with this older view, I am skeptical about any society's attempts to do something about dementia if they are not accompanied by an equally intense inquiry into ourselves. As many writers have pointed out, the activist impulse, divorced form self-criticism, easily leads to trouble. A family with Alzheimer's must tackle some concrete problems, but how they solve them matters less than that they learn to live with them—and each other.

DEALING WITH FEAR AND SHAME

This brings me to the last aspect of dementia which I wish to discuss: its ability to trigger fear and shame. Shame has been a much-neglected category in moral analysis. Part of the reason for the neglect lies in a popular view that there is something wrong with being ashamed. Many of us, at one time or another, took a deep bath in an ideology that suggested that there is "nothing to be ashamed of"; we associate shame with inhibitions, and inhibitions seem old-fashioned. But the capacity for shame is a central part of our humanity, as Carl Schneider has argued.

Shame refers to our reaction to the exposure of what should have been concealed. I am ashamed when my privacy has been violated, when certain aspects of myself are made visible to the public. Schneider distinguished what he calls shame as *discretion*—which *anticipates* the possibility of disclosure—from shame as *disgrace*—which *follows* the disclosure. He notes that shame is closely tied to the body and that it is an aesthetic category. We are ashamed of the unattractive, the ugly, that which calls attention to itself. Schneider suggests close connection between shame and death, noting that one of our words for shame is "mortification" (Schneider, 1977).

Dementia triggers shame in at least two different ways. The most obvious is the shame we feel at association with demented people, which makes us want to draw back and keep our distance. This reaction arises from the fact that we recognize ourselves, disgraced, in the demented person. Our self-control and self-possession stripped away, the incoherent flow of our minds is reflected and refracted in the speech or dumb silence of the demented. Obviously there are differences, but this shame is rooted in a recognition of a once and future self in the other. We are mortified and want to resist the identification. Recognition of this feeling in myself need not be bad, if it leads to a willingness to own the identification rather than retreat.

The second level of shame mentioned by Schneider is shame in advance, or the shame that leads to discretion. Sometimes people are able empathetically to recognize what would shame someone and to help them to "cover." Sensitive care for the demented may entail a great deal of covering, neither futile nor a waste of time. Rather, it is the deepest form of respect for dignity. The appearance of the patient and the surroundings matter (and it goes without saying that many of our institutions are not good at keeping up appearances).

Our images of the demented as sources of shame, or as beings who suffer in isolation, or as people who can be discounted reflect our images of ourselves. They show us the strengths and limits of what we value about our lives. I think we should recognize the dignity of the demented as part of our lives and the lives of those we love, and as refracted images of ourselves. Recognition is a moment in which we should forget our pretensions and forgive ourselves and them. Lear says in Shakespeare's play about him:

> Pray, do not mock me:
> I am a very foolish fond old man,
> Fourscore and upward, not an hour more nor less;
> And to deal plainly,
> I fear I am not in my perfect mind.
> Methinks I should know you, and know this man;
> Yet I am doubtful: for I am mainly ignorant
> What place this is; and all the skill I have
> Remembers not these garments; nor I know not
> Where I did lodge last night. Do not laugh at me;
> For, as I am a man, I think this lady
> To be my child Cordelia.
> You must bear with me:
> Pray you now, forget and forgive: I am old and
> foolish. (Craig, 1951, p. 1012)

REFERENCES

Boffey, P. (1985). Alzheimer's disease: families are bitter. *New York Times* (May 7):15.

Brozan, N. (1982). Coping with the travail of Alzheimer's disease. *New York Times* (November 19):Style Section, p. 1.

Craig, H., ed. (1951). *The Complete Works of Shakespeare, King Lear* (Act IV, Scene 7):983–1016. Chicago: Scott, Foresman and Co.

Engelhardt, H.T., Jr. (1986). *The Foundations of Bioethics*. New York: Oxford University Press.

Fletcher, J. (1954). *Morals and Medicine*. Princeton, N.J.: Princeton University Press.

Meyer, L. (1982a). A family stranger. *Washington Post* (January 9):A8.

Meyer, L. (1982b). Alzheimer's disease. *Washington Post* (January 8):A10.

Schneider, C.D. (1977). *Shame, Exposure and Privacy*. Boston: Beacon Press.

Smith, D.H. (1989). Suffering, medicine and Christian theology. In S. Lammers and A. Verhey, eds., *On Moral Medicine*, pp. 251–261. Grand Rapids, Mich.: William B. Eerdman's Publishing Co.

5

HUMAN DIGNITY, DEMENTIA, AND THE MORAL BASIS OF CAREGIVING

Richard J. Martin

Stephen G. Post

If we send the sick to hospital, the mentally sick to the mental hospital, the infirm to the Old People's Home, those with nervous complaints to the clinic, and difficult children to the reformatory, it is undoubtedly because they will be better cared for there. But it is also a little bit, whether or not we admit it, in order to remove from our sight these witnesses to human frailty. Civilized society does not like to see distress and poverty.

—Paul Tournier, *The Meaning of Persons*

The experience of dementia produces vulnerability. The demented individual is unable to independently perform daily functions necessary for sustenance. He or she lives in a state of risk for physical and emotional harm resulting from impairments in judgment or from the callousness of those who do not wish to witness human frailty. Dementia produces an inability to reasonably interpret the physical and social world and leaves the sufferer vulnerable to abuse. Hence, the impaired individual lives in a state of potential danger, regardless of whether the individual experiences the subjective feelings of fear.

CARING

Care is herein defined as those acts that intervene to minimize this vulnerability and compensate for dependency. There are other definitions of care. The philosopher Milton Mayeroff, in his classic phenomenological description of care, suggested this: "To care for another person, in the most significant sense, is to help him grow and actualize himself" (Mayeroff, 1971, p. 1). In caring, added Mayeroff, we "experience the other as having potentialities and the need to grow" (Mayeroff, 1971, p. 6). But with severely demented elderly people, the language of potential and growth does not apply in any obvious way, as it would in the case of a newborn, for instance. If this hope to see the other grow is essential for the caregiver's continued commitment, severely demented elderly persons are a serious challenge. Our definition of caring cannot, realistically, include growth and potentiality, as Mayeroff's does.

The current plethora of uses of the term *care* tends to confuse examination of the nature of dementia care with its moral underpinnings. Care, for example, is the descriptor used both when referring to the high-technology and economic conflicts of the health "care" industry and when describing the emotional bonds of an intimate relationship. Whereas much of the literature in biomedical ethics and aging focuses on "end of life" issues and the use of complex life-sustaining technologies, this chapter will focus on daily-life issues and the most complex life-sustaining phenomenon—another human being dedicated to maintaining "vital" functions and protecting both life and dignity.

The provision of supervision and compensation for another's deficit life skills (i.e., caregiving) can certainly be seen as a commodity comprising x number of hours, tasks performed, decisions made. In fact, while generally removed from discussions of "life-sustaining" technologies open to allocation/rationing strategies, caregiving is an expensive activity. Great time, money, and human burden are required to do for others what they cannot do for themselves—whether care is provided by kin, friend, or a professional. These resources are as amenable to economic forces and potential limitation as any other health care technology. Yet can analysis of care as a commodity adequately address the moral basis for care? How can we adequately capture the nature of the caring, the relationship, which exists between the caregiver and the care recipient?

Sally Gadow (1988), in her article "Covenant without Cure: Letting Go and Holding On in Chronic Illness," distinguished between curing (the provision of action directed toward the goal of recovery) and caring (the covenantal relationship that exists as an end unto itself). Caring is not doing for the other so that an outcome may be achieved. Rather, it is being for the other regardless of outcome. Caring exists within the present, not intertwined with prognostic notions of future recovery and cure. The inherent self-denial of the caregiver is spurred not by ideals of martyrdom, but rather by simple necessity. Caring is focused not toward what will be if certain actions are done, but rather on the fact that they must be done. As curing is the act of the Promethean hero who steals the fire of life from the hands of the gods, so caring is the act of Sisyphus, forever rolling the rock uphill, only to watch it fall again. While such actions are absurd from a utilitarian perspective, they are filled with meaning if examined in light of covenant and fidelity.

Caring, according to Gadow, is the process of entering another's vulnerability and brokenness by "breaking" oneself. In the absence of objective distance (often requiring a discarding of the professional objectivity so long enshrined in the medical model), mutual brokenness and intimacy nourish care. This mutual brokenness is most powerfully illustrated when the dependent functions are most intimate and often most mundane. The physical contact and lack of privacy in bathing, toileting, and dressing another, which are demeaning tasks in the model of cure, become bonds of covenant in the model of care. The emotional distance of curative efforts directed toward the amelioration of disease and historically controlled by the social status and power of educated professional men compares with the intimacy of care historically provided by woman committed in the bonds of affection, blood, or religious faith.

CARING IN DEMENTIA

Gadow emphasized the moral requirement of the caregiver to prevent the loss of the patient to the disease. Actions performed for the dependent individual which enhance the distance between caregiver and care recipient in their emphasis on power are suspect. This is a particularly difficult admonition in reference to dementia care. The very nature of dementia has been described as a loss of self. In dementia, the body organ for which compensation is needed is not an arm or leg, but the brain. The primary dependent function is not praxis, it is cogito. To our modern understanding, right or wrong, it is the self. The responsibilities of serving as another's brain require performing not only memory and language functions, but also functions of judgment and self-control. It is a responsibility of great power. Yet it is power, and the consequent distance between the powerful and the powerless, which Gadow emphasizes as potentially immoral. True caregiving for the demented individual entails the ability to exert this degree of power in the context of a relationship with both the premorbid self and the currently demented self.

Caregivers often thrive on relationships. Caring for others helps activate their caring in return. But the norm of reciprocity which is at least partly present in some caregiving has absolutely no place here. Of course, caregivers can pretend that certain meaningful responses and gestures of appreciation exist, and this may in some sense strengthen them. But the potential for relationship, like knowledge, is very limited. The severely demented elderly will often manifest an emotional presence replete with gaiety and even laughter, but generally this is directed to anyone and everyone, if it is directed at all.

Caregivers can thrive on a sense of accomplishment. They ordinarily can see the results of their work with the disabled victim of an accident who now can rise from the confines of the bed and chair. They can witness the impaired neonate who now plays with other children in the neighborhood. But these results do not apply to severely demented elderly people. Rather, successful caregiving for severely demented older persons results in what is not seen: the accident prevented, the nutrition maintained, the excrement kept from covering the care recipient's body. Only in this limited sense does the caregiver see what care amounts to, how it helps the dependent.

The caregiver for the severely demented patient must be a person of faith, who has faith in caring as a way of being in the world. He or she must have some trust that caring is a source of meaning in life, and then proceed with confidence into the domain of the nearly unknowable ones. The antithesis to this faith, and its only serious alternative, is the destruction of the radically infirm.

Dependence is a universal element of the human condition. In this age of emphasis on autonomy, rights, and freedoms, it is important to underscore our inherent dependence on other human beings. The character of dementia and its striking capacity to rob an individual of previously attained functional abilities should not cloud our recognition of dependence as a "premorbid" condition. Our own experiences of receiving vital, necessary care are often best viewed prior to discussions of the moral characteristics, duties, and limits of providing care. No other species demonstrates the protracted period of functional dependence of the human child. Born without the physical or cognitive abilities to satisfy basic needs—such as nourishment, shelter, and warmth—the human is by necessity dependent on others. Throughout life, our experience as flesh and blood is one of constant vulnerability. The impact of a single misplacement of genetic material in utero or a momentary lapse at the steering wheel demonstrates the fragile nature of our often presumed independence in decision-making and daily function.

Hence, as the need for care is universal, so the provision of that care is a part of the fabric of civilization. Caring for the dependent young, the infirm, and the aged is essential humanity, a biological reality tantamount to breath. It is the impact of that caregiving in light of societal context (the role of women, economic pressures, multigenerational families) which constitutes a "new" crisis to be examined.

As there are numerous degrees of dependence, there are numerous modes of providing care. The care of the individual suffering from dementia, such as Alzheimer's disease, is unique in its breadth and depth. The areas of dependence of an individual with dementia vary broadly with the level of cognitive and functional impairment. Early in the course of the dementing illness, such as Alzheimer's disease, care entails assistance with judgment regarding continuing to work, driving a car, cooking meals, or handling finances. As the disease progresses, the patient is in need of supervision, often at all times. In patients with mild to moderate impairment, the emotional difficulties of fear and depression are of great importance. Later in the disease, the patient becomes dependent in his or her ability to perform basic functions of dressing and hygiene. Initially the patient needs supervision, prompting, and cuing, later needing direct compensation. These dependencies are unique, not only to dementia, but even to each demented individual. The individual profile of cognitive strengths and weaknesses (such as memory, language, visuospatial abilities) relates to a unique array of functional difficulties with disparate needs for supervision or compensation.

Again, it must be noted that care for the demented individual is not just sustenance of the individual's body, but protection of the person. The values, choices, and dignity of the demented are also vulnerable to harm or neglect. The caregiver is the keeper of the psyche as well as the soma.

Other models of caregiving seem inadequate to guide the caregiver toward a role appropriate for dementia care. The moderately to severely impaired person with dementia demands supervision comparable to a 2-year-old child. Yet the previously competent adult with diminished cognitive abilities is certainly no toddler, and social interactions stemming from such a model would be characterized by disrespect, condescension, and excessive use of power. Furthermore, the traditional image of "bedside" care, appropriate to the physically infirm or frail elderly, is grossly inadequate. The gentle image of bedside attendance is incongruent with an otherwise strong man in his early 60s who is informing you from his own living room that he will indeed drive that car and intends to "get home." The moral boundaries of the classic beneficence for the willful ill are inadequate when one considers the degree of proxy decision-making, behavior control, and even frank coercion required for even one morning's care of the demented individual. Dressing a disabled person and transferring from bed to chair can be, as Gadow described, aesthetically beautiful—a "dance" of sorts. Yet the same dance with a patient who is ambulatory, agitated, and hell-bent on wandering out of the house is a vaudeville of pratfalls and pants around ankles. It is as ridiculous to view as it is physically exhausting and emotionally tragic to perform.

The disease of dementia, while typified in the losses to cognitive ability, also entails troublesome and sometimes dangerous behavioral/ psychiatric symptoms. The caregiver often assists with decisions in daily care needs in an environment of paranoid delusions ("What did you do with my money?"), hallucinations ("Did you see my mother this morning?"), and agitated bedtime disruptions ("I have to go to work now."). These symptoms are further complicated by the constant lack of clarity as to the demented person's insight into his or her own illness, and the common fluctuations in insight and abilities on a daily, even hourly, basis.

Furthermore, the experience of caregiving takes on additional depth when one considers the context of relationships between patients and caregivers. To deal with the indignities of demented behavior, often far disparate from the premorbid self, is particularly difficult for family members. To "lose" one's closest confidant and lover and yet to interact daily in the intimate physical life of that person is to experience a sense of isolation not only from one's spouse, but also from one's own past and imagined future. The physical and emotional demands of caregiving often fuse in the context of relationship with the impaired individual. To bathe the naked body of the person who neither recognizes nor trusts you is a difficult task; to bathe the naked body of the man to whom you have made love for forty-five years, who now neither recognizes nor trusts you, is heartbreaking. While this pain is unique to spousal caregivers, children (notably daughters, when referring to direct care) also experience emotional difficulties in caring for the parent they once knew. Often the unreflected and ambivalent feelings regarding one's family are stirred when caring for the demented parent. One need only imagine the sexual advances of a father who believes his daughter to be his wife, or the pain unlocked by a parent's accusation of maleficence toward a child attempting to balance the checkbook, to appreciate these feelings.

Conversely, it is important to recognize that the experience of caregiving is not universally a negative one. The burdens of time and energy are juxtaposed with the sense of meaning, purpose, and identity gained from caring. The experience of loyalty and competence gained from successfully learning new life skills can offset new demands, even when caring for the severely demented elderly. Caregivers identify feelings of self-satisfaction and increased self-respect related to the knowledge of successful fulfillment of responsibility and coping with the challenges of care (Horowitz, 1985). Research supports that many caregivers believe themselves to be doing a good job, having learned how to deal with a difficult situation (Pearlin et al., 1990; Lawton et al., 1989). In one study of dementia, care frustrations, and gratifications, spousal caregivers' well-being was more strongly related to the meaning ascribed to caregiving than the amount of care actually provided (Motenko, 1989). In this study, caregivers identified motives of reciprocity, responsibility, and desire to provide the most loving care as foremost factors providing meaning for their experience.

FAMILY CAREGIVERS

Elderly persons who need care have a strong preference for remaining in their homes and being cared for by friends or relatives. As of 1985, only 21 percent were in nursing homes (Rivlin and Wiener, 1988). Moreover, "nearly 90 percent of the disabled old people who were not in nursing homes received assistance from relatives and friends, sometimes supplemented by paid services. The majority of unpaid caregivers are women relatives of the disabled, usually wives, daughters, or daughters-in-law" (Rivlin and Wiener, 1988, p. 5). The gender factor is so striking that it is necessary to consider the basis and limits of family caregiving in a manner consistent with the fact that women do so much of the caring.

The image of "women in the middle" comes from the work of Elaine M. Brody, who has been a leading writer in the area of gerontology and the lives of modern women. Broadly defined, "women in the middle" are those who find themselves in the role of caregiving daughter while also fulfilling obligations to children and perhaps working for income (Brody, 1981). Circumstances can vary from individual to individual, but the image refers generally to those women who confront pressures of competing obligations which seem overwhelming. Brody asks whether younger and middle-aged women are now questioning their duties toward elderly parents in order to direct emotional and financial resources elsewhere.

Brody's main thesis is this: Despite the greatly accelerated rate of increase in the elderly population and the extent to which women find themselves placed in the role of primary caregiver, relatively younger and middle-aged women do not feel alienated from their elderly parents. Given the large-scale entry of women into the work force, it might be supposed that obligations to the old would be the first to suffer some erosion. The "role overload" that results from the pressure of juggling job, home, parenting, and care for the old might place obligations to elderly parents on thin ice. However, Brody marshals an impressive array of empirical evidence to support the following claim: "The vast majority of all three generations of women—the grandmothers, the daughters, and the young adult granddaughters—resoundingly endorsed the traditional value of filial responsibility to the aged. . . . Significantly, this traditional value held its ground among our middle-generation subjects even though 60% of them work" (Brody, 1981, p. 475). As a matter of fact, then, women do not appear to be discarding their sense of obligation to elderly parents despite demographic shifts and new pressures. Whether this level of commitment will be sustained in the future remains an open question.

According to Brody's studies, there is ample evidence that women want men to share equally in caring for elderly parents; but there is also clear evidence that women do most of the personal caring. Sons and husbands are likely to make financial commitments, but not emotionally demanding direct caring ones. They leave the latter to women. Thus, in reality, when appeals are made to family caregiving, this is often merely euphemism; it is "adult daughters (and daughters-in-law), who are the true alternatives" to nonfilial care (Brody, 1981, p. 474). Often it is women who are "assigned" the caregiver role with neither their consent nor their needs seriously considered.

Very quickly, then, the much vaunted "filial duties" become the imposed responsibility of daughters or daughters-in-law. The affective strain of physical caring is placed on women, while men are less directly involved—they might assist with financial management, funeral arrangements, and the like. Thus, the modern technological extension of the life span has put pressures most directly on women rather than on men.

Some women may have the affective resources and inclinations to shoulder this monumental responsibility; they may choose to live lives of significant self-abnegation, and they are free to do so. But heterogeneity among women deserves its due; many women will not want to make a vocation of caring for the cognitively impaired aged. Brody may be right in claiming that women still take obligations to aging parents seriously, but the new order of magnitude in this moral sphere brought about by the demographic transition, coupled with a male tendency to avoid direct caregiving, may alter the attitudes of women in the future.

Over the past several years, a number of philosophers have taken up the question of the basis of and limits to filial obligations. The late Jane English (1979) contributed an important essay entitled "What Do Grown Children Owe Their Parents?" Her response to the question is this: "I will contend that the answer is 'nothing' " (English, 1979, p. 351). This is because adult children do not "owe" anything to parents, but rather ought to care for their parents on the basis of genuine friendship or love. Parents, after all, are the ones who decide to have a child;

the child does not choose to be born and therefore has no obligations to parents based simply on her or his existence. Moreover, some parents abuse, neglect, and in other ways seriously harm their child; others benefit their child only in the most minimal fashion and are willing to sacrifice very little, if at all. These realities pressed English to reconstruct the question of how adult children are to relate morally to their parents through an appeal to reciprocity in the context of friendship. If parents genuinely care for their child, mutual beneficence ought to be the norm, and English encouraged this ideal. However, when friendship is absent, the demands of reciprocity are absent as well.

This position is clearly revisionist; whereas tradition emphasized "filial obligations" that could easily lead to the exploitation of daughters, English suggested an alternative vision. While we might want to give more attention to past friendship than did English, and even to a limited use of the language of "obligation" and "owe," her position responds to a valid interest in protecting young and adult children against unfair filial obligations. D. Lydia Bronte pointed out that in the 1940s and 1950s, some parents in certain sections of the United States practiced a form of familial slavery. A daughter, viewed as mere "property" by her parents, could be forced to remain at home and unmarried in order to serve as their designated care "giver." With reference to rural Arkansas several decades ago, Bronte says that some daughters rebelled and married against parental wishes, but a number of these suffered emotional breakdowns due to the anger and vindictiveness of parents (Bronte, 1988). Filial obligation or debt, then, can serve as a maleficent ideological warrant for the destruction of daughters. There is no reason to think that this kind of harm to daughters has not been a frequent problem in certain regions of the United States and the world.

Appeals to filial obligations are immediately suspect from a feminist perspective. English made an important contribution to contemporary feminist moral thought because she articulated this suspicion. There is, though, a restoration of filial obligations offered by Christina Hoff Sommers.

Sommers was specifically critical of English because the latter "denies outright that there are any filial obligations not grounded in mutual friendship" (Sommers, 1986, p. 439). English, claimed Sommers, focused too narrowly on examples of unworthy parents, while ignoring "what is owed to the average parent who is neglected or whose wishes are disregarded when they could at some reasonable cost be respected" (Sommers, 1986, p. 441). While Sommers was willing to acknowledge that "exceptional parents can forfeit their moral claims on their children," she was most concerned with morally unwarranted disregard for filial obligations. While Sommers considered suspicion of filial obligations, she was unwilling to radically diminish their weight. Sommers proposed a retrieval of filial obligations based on the notion of gratitude—a gratitude both for the gift of life and for the care bestowed in childhood. There are morally valid expectations rooted in the principle of reciprocity and the unique quality of the parent-child interrelationship which have as their first line of defense the wider historical tradition of Western ethics. Embedded within tradition is the recognition that reciprocity remains valid as the norm of intergenerational morality despite the expected failures of both children and parents to manifest a consistent generosity. Moreover, the fact that a child does not determine her or his own birth failed to convince Sommers that the gift of life has no reciprocal pull based on gratitude. Furthermore, Sommers observed, most people do feel obligated to their parents, so English departed from "common sense" and the wisdom of the ordinary person's moral sensibilities. She ended by expressing concern with the moral chaos that would likely result from any radical revisionism prepared to suspend filial obligations generally considered. It must be emphasized that Sommers did not think filial obligations hold when parents fail to uphold accepted child-rearing standards; she simply focused on the ordinary circumstances rather than the exceptional.

Though there are similarities between English and Sommers in that both appeal to the idea of reciprocity, the disparity between their views is considerable due to disagreement over what reciprocity encompasses. With regard to English, reciprocity pertains only to the *present*, whereas Sommers looked back in time and considered the requital due *past* beneficence.

It may well be that Sommers' more traditional view still defines the perspective of women, as Brody suggests; however, the suspicions of English may become more dominant not so much because more parents fail their children but rather because the caregiving demands of the elderly are gradually becoming so much greater than ever before as the "success" of medicine has extended life as well as chronic illness. Pollster Daniel Yankelovich, cited in Callahan (1987, p. 13), claims that grown children now feel that they owe their parents less than was the case a generation ago. As the potential for responsibility for a demented parent, a drug-impaired child, or an economically damaged household increases, it is likely that the problem of competing obligations for the "woman in the middle" would intensify. Filial obligations could give way to rationing health care on the basis of age, and even to a policy of "direct termination" of the elderly as advocated by philosopher Margaret P. Battin (1987). Precisely how the status of filial obligation might change in the future is an open question, and one that will increasingly command our philosophical attention.

In the context of an aging society, the heterogeneity of women must be stressed in order to avoid patriarchal manipulation of "relational feminism." This school of thought, as recently assessed by Deborah L. Rhode (1988), stresses the importance of relationships and caregiving traits to women. The diversity of women, cautions Rhode, may be obscured as a result, and a homogenized "woman's perspective" could result. It is important, argues Rhode, not to understate the heterogeneity of women.

FROM FILIAL TO GENERAL DUTIES

There was recently an extraordinary case that presented at a university geriatric clinic. A particular woman brought her markedly demented father to the clinic for medical, nursing, and social service attention— the father who had sexually molested her for many years. She did not live with him, nor did she have any correspondence with him. But when she learned from a sibling that he needed help and that others were unwilling to assist, she brought him for care. She had every right to relinquish all caring for her father, who had so utterly failed her. Yet, as she put it, despite the fact that she could not care for him as a father, she could at least care for him as a stranger, as one human being among slews of others who, despite their grievous faults, are worthy of respect simply as human beings.

Here the moral shift was from the domain of special relations to the domain of strangers, to humans qua humans. It is, of course, difficult to see caring as a central activity when the one cared for is a stranger. Such insight requires a rather dramatic break from dominant images of human fulfillment which characterize a laissez-faire culture. Caring does not draw on the competitive spirit, or on ambition unleashed. It has nothing to do with the equality of opportunity which defines fairness in the race for success. It requires a form of individualism which resists certain concepts of the normal and which views the extrinsically unrewarded activities of caring as intrinsically rewarding. This is supported by consideration of the low social status and monetary compensation often given to those nonkin who directly care for the demented elderly in private homes, day care, and nursing homes. These minimally educated caregivers are, in fact, delegated huge responsibility for the protection of another's being—all for compensation marginally above minimum wage. These caregivers face, and necessarily resolve, the dilemmas—such as proxy decision-making and use of coercion— which we in the professional community continue to debate.

A major emphasis of the current public policy debate regarding dementia, most easily recognized in discussion of advance directives and "living wills," is the relationship between the predemented self and the "shell" of that self left since the progression of dementia. These are constructs and metaphors not often expressed by nursing assistants. For the nonfilial caregiver, such as the nursing assistant, the demented self is truly the person. Generally, the past personality and accomplishments of the demented patient are unknown or moot. The emotional bonds built between care provider and patient, bonds as deep and varied as any with a cognitively intact patient, are based in the present reality. The relationships built with the moderately to severely demented are neither embellished nor encumbered by a past history of reciprocal love or hate. They are relationships of moments; as memory is not expected, each interaction is the true test of commitment, trust, and caring.

Mary Howell (1984, p. 657) contrasted the experience of nursing attendants for the demented elderly with that of family members who can make a distinction in perspective between the current relationship with the "person who is" and a past relationship with the "person who was." This contrast is particularly important when one considers how little influence the current nonfilial care provider has in formal decision-making regarding the demented individual's care. While the nursing attendant has incredible power over the daily life of this person for whom he or she may provide care, it is predominantly those most invested in the "person who was" who will decide about life-sustaining treatment, food and fluid support, and similar matters.

The pressing need of caring for the increasing number of demented elderly people demands that, given current care technology and legal constraints regarding euthanasia, the competent nursing attendant will become more valued by our society. Whether that demand will translate to increased compensation may be left to economists to discuss. Hopefully the gerontological research community will increase its efforts toward study of the nonfilial direct care provider. Currently the psychological characteristics and moral reasoning of the nonfilial direct care provider are little studied and poorly understood. Anecdotal and journalistic reports of abuse and neglect by care attendants abound. Certainly the vulnerability of the demented elderly and the frequency of violent crime in our society should encourage us to make every effort to identify, eliminate, and prevent such occurrences. Yet it is particularly the competent, caring attendant of whom we know so little. Howell identified seven characteristics:

Among those who do this work well and with a sense of joy and accomplishment, I see these resources:

1. A belief in the value of every living person.
2. A willingness to become engaged and attached, not holding patients at a "clinical" or "objective" distance.
3. A deep pleasure and satisfaction in the skillful performance of complex and simple caretaking responsibilities—from making judgments about the promotion of well-being to the performance of the most elemental acts of intimate physical care.
4. An awareness and enjoyment of staff interactions—not only when they proceed smoothly and with comfortable communion, but also when they become scratchy and need to be worked on.
5. A tendency to unify individual and group energies in mobilization against a perceived "common enemy": all those who do not do this work, do not know how wearying it is, do not experience its urgencies and needs, and who treat staff and patients with either neglect or abuse.
6. A conviction—contrary to the conventional wisdom of medical professionalism—that this job is worth doing.
7. An enduring and compassionate sense of humor. (Howell, 1984, p. 658)

As stated previously, true caring for a stranger may require a special form of individualism, self-concept, and ego strength. Conversely, caring may require a communal ethic that ascribes to the care recipient a dignity independent of societal values of productivity or righteousness. In his study of Burmese Buddhist society, Daw Khin Myo Chit (1989) pointed out that even when elders are not deserving of respect and care, the norms of righteousness and noninjury still hold. "One of the things Buddhism teaches is not to react to people's frailties with one's own viciousness; in other words, you should not let the other's imperfections decide your conduct, for then you are not in command of yourself" (Daw Khin Myo Chit, 1989, p. 45).

Likewise, the Judeo-Christian tradition strongly emphasizes a value for the human individual independent of abilities and potential but rooted in the dignity bestowed upon the creature by the Creator. Caring may communicate less of the relationship between the care provider and the patient than of the relationship between the care provider and God. As recorded by the apostle Matthew, Jesus of Nazareth emphasized this principle: "Truly I say to you, as you did it not to one of the least of these, you did it not to me." Dr. Howell alluded to this principle and proposes a communal role of the care provider equally true of those who care for kin or stranger: "I, for one, believe that a significant measure of our humanity as a society is found in the kind of care given to patients such as the demented elderly. Those who care for 'the least of these' are carrying a burden that we might share in more fully. These caretakers deserve our expressed appreciation, at the very least" (Howell, 1984, p. 659).

REFERENCES

Battin, M.P. (1987). Age rationing and the just distribution of health care: is there a duty to die? In T.M. Smeeding, ed., *Should Medical Care Be Rationed by Age?* pp. 89–94. Totowa, N.J.: Rowman and Littlefield.

Brody, E. (1981). Women in the middle. *Gerontologist, 21:*471–480.

Bronte, D.L. Personal communication, September 14, 1988.

Callahan, D. (1987). *Setting Limits: Medical Goals in an Aging Society.* New York: Simon and Schuster.

Daw Khin Myo Chit. (1989). Add years to your life the Buddhist way. In W.M. Clements, ed., *Religion, Aging, and Health: A Global Perspective,* pp. 39–57. New York: Haworth Press.

English, J. (1979). What do grown children owe their parents? In O. O'Neill and W. Ruddick, eds., *Having Children: Philosophical and Legal Reflections on Parenthood,* pp. 351–356. New York: Oxford University Press.

Gadow, S. (1988). Covenant without cure: letting go and holding on in chronic illness. In J. Watson and M.A. Ray, eds., *The Ethics of Care and the Ethics of Cure: Synthesis in Chronicity,* pp. 5–14. New York: National League for Nursing.

Horowitz, A. (1985). Family caregiving to the frail elderly. In C. Eisdorfer, ed., *Annual Review of Gerontology and Geriatrics,* Vol. 5, pp. 194–246. New York: Springer Publishing Co.

Howell, M. (1984). Caretakers' views on responsibilities for the care of the demented elderly. *Journal of the American Geriatrics Society, 32(9):*657–660.

Lawton, M.P., Kleban, M.H., Moss, M., Ravine, M., and Glicksman, A. (1989). Measuring caregiver appraisal. *Journal of Gerontology: Psychological Sciences, 44:*61–71.

Mayeroff, M. (1971). *On Caring.* New York: Harper and Row.

Motenko, A.K. (1989). The frustrations, gratifications, and well-being of dementia caregivers. *Gerontologist, 29:*166–172.

Pearlin, L.I., Mullin, J.T., Semple, S.J., and Skaff, M.M. (1990). Caregiving and the stress process: an overview of concepts and their measures. *Gerontologist, 30:*583–591.

Rhode, D.L. (1988). The "women's point of view." *Journal of Legal Education, 38:*39–46.

Rivlin, A.M., and Wiener, J.M. (1988). *Caring for the Disabled Elderly: Who Will Pay?* Washington, D.C.: Brookings Institution.

Sommers, C.H. (1986). Filial morality. *Journal of Philosophy, 83:*439–456.

Tournier, P. (1957). *The Meaning of Persons.* New York: Harper and Row.

PART II. Treatment Decisions, Advance Directives, and Euthanasia

6

AUTONOMY REVISITED: THE LIMITS OF ANTICIPATORY CHOICES

Rebecca S. Dresser

As the health of dementia patients declines, those who love and care for them may face decisions on the level of life-sustaining treatment these patients should receive. Although the most frequent questions concern resuscitation efforts, they can also concern provision of antibiotics, dialysis, surgery, medical nutrition and hydration, and other treatment modalities. Because most dementia patients are incapable of making informed treatment decisions for themselves, such decisions fall to family members, caregivers, and others. What standards should guide these proxy decision-makers in their struggle to make morally defensible choices?

In my view, the standards articulated thus far by ethicists, courts, and policymakers are inadequate, conceptually confused, and morally problematic. According to the accepted approach, treatment choices on behalf of incompetent patients—those who are unable to choose for themselves—should incorporate whatever relevant preferences and values the patient expressed while competent; that is, treatment should be what the patient "would want" if competent to choose. The underlying assumption is that the competent individual's concept of personal well-being applies equally to the patient as a demented person. Yet this assumption is vulnerable to challenge, for in significant respects the demented patient is no longer the one who formerly expressed the treatment preferences. Indeed, the patient's well-being now could be quite different from that of the former competent person.

In this chapter, I analyze and criticize the accepted approach to decision-making for incompetent patients and offer an alternative approach to resolving these decisions. With a few exceptions, treatment decisions made according to the accepted approach have not departed from those my alternative approach would produce. My concern is with the reasoning implicit in the accepted approach, which creates the possibility of future disturbing outcomes, particularly regarding conscious demented patients who retain the ability to interact with their environments. In the first part of the chapter, I review the dominant approach to treatment decision-making evident in court decisions and other sources. The second part is a discussion of this "subjective" approach and its inherent problems. Part three includes an analysis of "objective" or "best interests" treatment standards. Next I compare the moral implications of the two approaches. I then discuss the discretion that proxy decision-makers have been accorded under the subjective approach. The chapter concludes with an argument on the need to formulate societal judgments on the boundaries of acceptable treatment decisions for demented patients.

THE CONVENTIONAL APPROACH TO TREATMENT DECISION-MAKING

Beginning with *In re Quinlan* (1976), the courts and other legal decision-makers have shown a marked preference for what is generally labeled the subjective, or substituted judgment, approach. This preference is evident in the dominant trend in the case law, as well as the numerous living-will and other advance-directive statutes enacted by state legislatures (Weir, 1989). The goal of this approach is, briefly stated, to resolve treatment dilemmas the same way the individual patients would if they were competent. As the decision in the case of *In re Jobes* put it, "the patient's right to self-determination is the guiding principle in determining whether to continue or withdraw life-sustaining treatment; . . . therefore the goal of a surrogate decision-maker for an incompetent patient must be to determine and effectuate what that patient, if competent, would want" (1987, 529 A.2d, pp. 436–437).

This approach builds on the competent patient's nearly absolute legal right to decide whether or not to accept life-prolonging medical interventions. Legal decision-makers have reasoned that if incompetent patients are to receive equal respect, then they must be given this right as well (Dresser and Robertson, 1989).

Incompetent patients cannot choose which treatment course they would prefer, however. To fill this information void, the customary move is to look to evidence of incompetent patients' former statements and behavior indicating the treatment preferences they had as competent persons. This evidence may be in the form of an explict oral or written treatment directive, such as a living will, less formal statements made to friends and family, or more general information about a patient's attitudes toward life and medical treatment, such as past hospital decisions, religious beliefs, and character traits.

This approach has yielded numerous court decisions permitting life-sustaining treatment to be withheld or withdrawn from terminally ill, permanently unconscious, and severely demented incompetent patients (Weir, 1989). More recently, however, it has also led a few courts to order treatment continued for such patients. In these cases, courts applying strict evidentiary standards determined that there was insufficient information to establish that the patients would refuse the treatment if they were competent. In the absence of such evidence, treatment had to continue, despite the claims of families and others that these patients failed to obtain benefits from this treatment (*Cruzan v. Harmon*, 1989; *In re Westchester County Medical Center*, 1988; *Evans v. Bellevue Hospital*, 1987).

THE SUBJECTIVE APPROACH—ITS NATURE AND LIMITATIONS

The subjective approach begins with the judgment that autonomy is a value to be promoted whenever possible. Autonomy is a good thing because it tends to advance individual welfare, given that we generally know how to further our own interests better than anyone else does (Buchanan and Brock, 1986). In addition, respecting autonomy allows us as individuals to shape our lives "according to some coherent and distinctive sense of character, conviction, and interest" (Dworkin, 1986, p. 8). Except for a few unusual situations, then, even when competent persons' choices fail to advance their best interests, we should not interfere with those choices. Thus, treatment decisions about life and death should virtually always lie in the hands of the individual patient, who must experience the consequences of the choice.

But how can autonomous decision-making exist if the patient is permanently unconscious, demented, or otherwise unable to understand the information relevant to a treatment decision? Contemporaneous autonomy obviously is impossible in such cases. Without much analysis, courts and other decision-makers have automatically embraced what Ronald Dworkin calls "precedent autonomy" as the replacement (p. 10). Thus, any former statements, behavior, and so forth representing the patient's competent beliefs relevant to the current treatment issue should govern the outcome.

Although the legal sources fail to provide justification for this move, philosophers and other commentators have sought to do so. For example, Ronald Dworkin argues that if we genuinely respect autonomy, we should let prior choices govern future treatment. He acknowledges that even the competent person's carefully considered statements about future life-sustaining treatment are not as informed as we would like them to be, given that the person has usually never faced the actual situation presenting the need for a choice. There is always the possibility that a person's preferences would be different when actually coping with that situation. But Dworkin contends that true respect for autonomy means prior choices should control future treatment, even if those choices are detrimental to the incompetent patient's current well-being. Indeed, they should be implemented even if the now-demented patient explicitly expresses different wishes, perhaps asking for treatment that was refused in a living will (p. 130). According to Dworkin, failing to do so denies people the power to shape the whole of their lives as they wish to, which is a crucial dimension of their autonomy (p. 13). Nancy Rhoden also took this view in arguing that the law should empower competent persons to reflect on their histories, values, and relationships and make the future treatment decisions that most harmonize with these considerations (Rhoden, 1988).

But even Dworkin admits that there may be good reasons to violate precedent autonomy, such as to avoid inhumane denials of life-sustaining treatment. Similarly, Rhoden agreed that there should be an exception to the general rule requiring adherence to advance directives if they would produce the death of mildly demented, "pleasantly senile" patients (Rhoden, 1990). Allen Buchanan, another strong supporter of advance directives, acknowledges that they might justifiably be overridden to protect an incompetent patient's welfare (Buchanan, 1988).

In sum, I make three cautionary points about precedent autonomy. First, because precedent autonomy is typically directed toward a future situation that the individual has never confronted, its expression may not be what that person would in reality choose. Thus, an exercise of precedent autonomy might carry less weight than a contemporaneous autonomous choice. Second, autonomy is not the sole value relevant to treatment decision-making, and it could permissibly be limited in some cases to protect other values. Finally, in most treatment dilemmas concerning incompetent patients, there has been no exercise of precedent autonomy. When proxy decision-makers reflect on a patient's former informal remarks, general attitudes about medical treatment, character traits, and so forth, to determine what the patient "would want," autonomy is not involved (Dworkin, 1986, p. 14; Rhoden, 1988, pp. 388–396). As Nancy Rhoden put it, "proxies can implement a patient's right to privacy, which has come to mean a right to make an autonomous choice, only when the patient has in fact made a prior choice. In other cases, although proxy decisions may humanely look to such concerns as the patient's [former] interests or probable preferences, they do not, properly speaking, implement the patient's right to choose, because the patient has made no actual choice" (1988, p. 377). Although it may be morally defensible to incorporate general information about a patient's former concerns into the decision process, this information should not be accorded the same compelling weight as an exercise of precedent autonomy (Ellman, 1990).

OBJECTIVE TREATMENT STANDARDS

Objective, or "best interests," treatment standards are an alternative to the subjective approach. The New Jersey Supreme Court in the case of *In re Conroy* (1985 [hereafter *Conroy*, 1985]) held that nontreatment of a severely demented patient would be permissible if "the net burdens of the patient's life with the treatment . . . clearly and markedly outweigh the benefits that the patient derives from life" and "the recurring, unavoidable and severe pain of the patient's life [is] such that the effect of administering life-sustaining treatment would be inhumane" (98 N.J. p. 365, 486 A.2d p. 1232). In *Barber v. Superior Court* (1983), the court asserted that decisions should be guided by a determination of whether the proposed treatment is proportionate or disproportionate in terms of the benefit to be gained versus the burden imposed.

These tests contemplate a focus on the incompetent patient's current condition, together with an assessment of the benefits and burdens that administering or forgoing treatment would entail for that patient. Treatment decisions thus reflect the patient's interests as an incompetent person. Instead of looking to a patient's living will or other exercise of precedent autonomy to determine whether or not to treat, decision-makers consider what choice would best protect the patient as an incompetent person. This is frequently the approach used to resolve treatment dilemmas involving children, as well as retarded adults who never were capable of exercising autonomy (Weir, 1989, pp. 157–158).

It is important to understand how the interests of demented patients might differ from those they had as competent persons. The treatment preferences of competent persons reflect what matters to them as competent individuals, including work and other mental challenges, physical mobility, and a network of complex social relationships. When life-prolonging treatment would bring about conditions that would unacceptably intrude on the values that they hold dear, and the activities that make life worth living for them, then competent patients decide against treatment. But when people become demented and physically debilitated, what was once important to them often is forgotten, while physical comfort and what we might view as low-level interactions with people and their environments often become vitally significant. In general, competent people have the opportunity to alter their important personal choices, within certain limits created by their obligations to others. But incompetent patients lose the chance to change their minds about their treatment, and some could be seriously harmed by decisions to treat them in accord with their former wishes (Dresser and Robertson, 1989; Dresser, 1990).

What interests do demented patients have which might shape treatment decisions? The objective approach seeks to identify the features of any human life which count as benefits and burdens, and to weigh them as they apply to an individual patient (Rhoden, 1988, p. 398). (This second step of individualization means that even "objective" treatment standards have a subjective component, in that they are concerned with how each patient experiences life.) The *Conroy* court discussed physical, emotional, and intellectual experiences as relevant factors (1985, 98 N.J. pp. 365–367). Thus, a conscious demented patient facing a future of unremediable pain, without any countervailing positive experiences, need not be treated. Conversely, the mildly demented patient needing a relatively unintrusive medical intervention must receive it.

The *Conroy* objective test falls short, however, when it is applied to permanently unconscious patients. *Conroy* held that treatment may be forgone only when severe, uncontrollable pain outweighs any benefit the patient obtains from life (1985, 98 N.J. pp. 365–367). Permanently unconscious patients fail to experience pain or other physical sensations, according to existing medical knowledge. Thus the burdens of treatment and continued life cannot be "inhumane" to such patients. Must they be treated, then, even though their lack of consciousness also prevents them from obtaining any benefit from continued life? In my view, the objective test should permit nontreatment in such cases, because permanently unconscious patients themselves lack significant interests in having their lives continued. Because they are completely unable to interact with anyone or anything in their environment, life can hold no meaning for them. A decision to forgo life-sustaining treatment thus cannot harm them in any morally significant way (see President's Commission for the Study of Ethical Problems in Medicine and Biomedical and Behavioral Research, 1983, pp. 182–183, 186).

A similar argument can be made regarding the "barely conscious" patient. At some point, patients may become so severely demented that their lives consist simply of, as John Arras described it, "being there" (Arras, 1984, p. 31). Although capable of experiencing some physical sensations, they make no purposeful movements and lack the cognitive capacity to interact with the environment. Again, even if treatment entails little physical burden, it is hard to see what these patients gain from continued life in such states. As Nancy Rhoden argued, mere consciousness, like biological life, is not a morally significant end in itself. Instead, it is a necessary condition for achieving the ends that *are* of moral value to us—thought, emotion, pleasure, and relationships with the world (Rhoden, 1985, p. 1320).

On the other hand, many mildly or moderately demented patients do appear to obtain significant benefits from continued life. Although these benefits may seem small to us, we must evaluate them from the patients' perspectives, recognizing that they cannot now experience the wealth of our lives as competent persons and that they are usually unaware that they have lost the more complex existence they once enjoyed (Arras, 1984, p. 30). Given their limits, then, patients who can relate to the people and objects surrounding them typically have lives that for them are significantly better than no life at all. As one caregiver described her patients:

> We have often heard of our demented elderly patients "the person is absent" or "gone." . . . Relatives of patients, reflecting on changes they see in personality, cognitive abilities, and relationships, grieve for their own sense of loss, their awareness of what is no longer.
>
> But for anyone who gives direct care, each patient is at the same time fully a person, of spirit and body both. Although Mr. X is different from the person he once was, and to those who knew him in past years, may seem to be "less" of a person, to those who care for him day by day, he is a fulsome and substantial person, indeed. He requires care that is thoughtfully planned and executed; his social relationships are complex, difficult and often unpredictable—just as might be said of any of us—and his immediate needs range from those related to bare survival to remnants of mature and sophisticated development represented, for instance, by the enjoyment of music. (Howell, 1984, p. 657)

One common criticism of objective treatment standards is that outside observers simply cannot "objectively" evaluate a patient's interests. It is impossible for others to assume either the exact position of the patient or a thoroughly neutral position apart from their own subjective views (Nagel, 1986). Hence, it is an illusion to believe that objective tests can supplant subjective treatment standards. I have two responses to this criticism. First, current work in the philosophy of mind and in artificial intelligence counters the above mystical approach to human consciousness, contending instead that it is possible to attain an objective understanding of how another person experiences the world (Dennett, 1987). Second, we live our lives as if we *can* know the mental states of other human beings, competent and incompetent. By observing and interpreting their behavior, which may or may not include language, we impute mental states to other people, including infants and retarded individuals (see Dennett, 1987, pp. 43–57). Such "folk psychology" may be inaccurate and in need of refinement, especially as people become less and less "like us." But I think we can understand, and get better at understanding, enough about the worlds of incompetent patients to arrive at rough judgments on what life is like for them, as well as on the burdens and benefits treatment would entail.

Objective treatment standards, then, focus on the individual the demented patient is now, rather than the competent person the patient once was. In addition, it should be recognized that because it is the incompetent patient who will bear the burdens and enjoy the benefits of a treatment decision, that decision rests on what currently matters to the patient, rather than what was important to the patient as a competent person.

MORAL IMPLICATIONS OF SUBJECTIVE AND OBJECTIVE STANDARDS

The choice between subjective and objective treatment standards has inescapable, but largely unrecognized, moral implications. If precedent autonomy controls decision-making for incompetent patients, moral priority is given to the desires of competent persons to protect their own interests. Accordingly, competent persons who find even mild dementia "degrading and without human dignity" may direct that antibiotic treatment be withheld if they become cognitively impaired and contract pneumonia, despite their apparently pleasant lives as mildly impaired individuals (*Brophy v. New England Sinai Hospital*, 1986). Likewise, the competent "vitalists" who strongly value all biological life may choose the most aggressive measures to delay death, even if such care becomes painful, distressing, and obviously futile for them as terminally ill incompetent patients (*In re Conroy*, 1985, 98 N.J. pp. 366–367). Protection thus is given to the competent person's concerns about the future, rather than to the welfare of the incompetent patient that person subsequently becomes.

A policy choice in favor of the subjective treatment standard says, in effect, that we accord greater moral value to the precedent autonomy of a moral agent than to the welfare of an individual incapable of exercising autonomy (Rhoden, 1988). Thus, it is better to harm the demented incompetent patient by effectuating an advance directive than to harm the competent person by disregarding that person's exercise of precedent autonomy. Incompetent patients may justifiably be subjected to treatment decisions that fail to serve their interests, so that competent persons may have the future control they seek.

I put the conflict so starkly to illustrate the hidden bias inherent in the subjective approach to treatment decision-making. It is not surprising that policymakers, perhaps inadvertently, have adopted this approach. First, those contemplating the issue, as individuals and as policymakers, are competent persons. Understandably, such persons give great weight to the wish for future control to safeguard their present values and concerns. But it does not follow that this view represents the appropriate moral stance. In our contemporary culture, we allegedly believe that individuals who lack the full range of normal human capacities ought to receive protection and assistance, so that their lives may be as full as is possible for them. Adhering to this ideal in the treatment context requires us to recognize our current bias, and seek to mitigate it (Dresser, 1990, p. 433).

Second, in the vast majority of cases, competent persons do not intend to order decisions that would conflict with their future well-being. The relatively few individuals who make explicit advance directives usually are concerned with avoiding treatment when terminal illness becomes significantly debilitating, or when permanent unconsciousness or severe dementia destroys their ability to interact with the world. Those persons who express their competent treatment preferences more informally sound a similar note to those who make explicit directives. Indeed, perhaps the most frequently made assertion is: "I don't want to be a vegetable like Karen Quinlan." As I argued earlier, nontreatment under such circumstances fails to harm the incompetent patient. Overbroad language in a patient's prior statements, however, may inadvertently authorize nontreatment when treatment would materially benefit the patient. Respect for precedent autonomy does not require that such statements be so construed, because they do not represent an informed choice. Yet the subjective approach to treatment decision-making creates the possibility for nontreatment in these circumstances.

I believe we need a more explicit focus on the incompetent patient. Although such patients are incapable of moral agency, they may retain significant interests in having their lives continue. Such an existence has moral value, despite the lack of moral agency. Precedent autonomy should be limited, in my view, so that the welfare of such patients may be protected. The competent person's interest in ordering future care that is seriously detrimental to that individual as an incompetent patient is less morally compelling than the incompetent patient's interest in protection from substantial harm. The limit on precedent autonomy is also needed, I submit, to meet society's interest in protecting a meaningful sense of respect for human life. As a result, the mildly demented patient enjoying what we as competent persons perceive as simple pleasures ought to be treated, as long as the treatment itself fails to entail substantial burdens. Similarly, the former vitalist suffering uncontrollable pain and distress from intensive care that can preserve life for only a few weeks should be allowed a comfortable death. Such choices are integral to maintaining our society's purported moral concern for vulnerable, disabled individuals.

PROXY DISCRETION IN TREATMENT DECISION-MAKING

In most cases involving life-sustaining treatment for incompetent patients, there has been no exercise of precedent autonomy. It is therefore perhaps even more important to confront the conceptual and moral issues raised in these cases. Unfortunately, many courts have spoken in terms of autonomy and self-determination rights in cases in which there are only very vague and largely indeterminate indications of what the patient "would want." A few courts have even imposed the autonomy model on cases involving patients who *never* were competent (Rhoden, 1988, pp. 385–388)!

Another common judicial device has been to refer to the interests incompetent patients, including permanently unconscious patients, have in such matters as privacy, dignity, and bodily integrity. While it is true that less seriously impaired patients may have rudimentary interests of this nature, the courts have failed to realize that such interests are not necessarily possessed by incompetent patients as a group. The clearest example is the permanently unconscious patient, who completely lacks awareness of the environment and simply cannot now have any of these concerns. The courts have failed to recognize the difference between *imputing* such concerns to patients, versus determining that they matter to a particular individual patient who has the capacities necessary to appreciate and value privacy, dignity, and bodily integrity. If incompetent patients themselves cannot appreciate these concerns, they should not be attributed to the patients. When privacy, dignity, and bodily integrity are factors in these cases, they actually refer to interests the patient may have had as a competent person, or to the beliefs family members, health care professionals, and the broader society have about how to respect such values in the treatment of incompetent patients (Dresser, 1988).

In short, courts applying the accepted approach to treatment decision-making have created a conceptual muddle in which respect for incompetent patients' "autonomy" often represents very different considerations. In addition, the approach yields a focus either on the patient in a former competent state or on a hypothetical "reasonable person," rather than on the incompetent patient whose treatment is at issue. The imprecision entailed in determining what the incompetent patient "would want" opens the door to distortion, and decisions may end up resting on a family's or other observer's distress at seeing the patient in a deteriorated condition, or on financial considerations.

The phenomenon is evident in two Massachusetts cases involving conscious incompetent patients. *In re Spring* (1980 [hereafter *Spring*, 1980]) involved a demented nursing home patient in his late 70s who needed renal dialysis to survive but had no other serious health problems. At times, he physically resisted the dialysis and was sedated for the procedure. The patient's wife and son eventually sought a court order authorizing termination of the dialysis. The court granted their request, based on the family's claim that if the patient were competent, he would refuse the dialysis. The relatives failed to present any evidence of the patient's specific or general treatment preferences relevant to the situation, but claimed that his former physically active life-style indicated that he would refuse treatment if he were competent.

The *Spring* court thus handled the case as if the patient retained the concerns he once had. As a result, it failed to inquire into the patient's present life experiences. Thus it did not know whether he enjoyed various activities and interactions, whether he was physically comfortable except during dialysis, or if behavior modification or other interventions had been attempted as a means of improving his attitude toward dialysis. To protect Spring's welfare as an incompetent patient, the court needed to assess whether he would enjoy benefits from continued life which would outweight his periodic irritation with dialysis and whether the burdens he experienced from dialysis could be reduced. Instead, the court and the patient's family concentrated on what some (certainly not all) competent people in the patient's situation would choose, ignoring this specific patient's contemporaneous welfare. Moreover, the court failed to take into account the possibility that the family's own distress and financial concerns influenced their views of what Spring "would want" in this situation, issuing a decision that may have been detrimental to this patient's material interests in obtaining life-sustaining treatment.

A second instance of conceptually inappropriate analysis occurred in *In re Hier* (1984 [hereafter *Hier*, 1984]), which involved a demented elderly woman who had been institutionalized since her 30s for psychiatric reasons. Several years before the case arose, she had been given a gastrostomy tube for a physical problem that impaired her ability to ingest food orally. She apparently had no other health problems. The court case arose when she pulled out the tube and covered the opening with her hands whenever doctors attempted to reinsert the tube. By the time the nursing home in which she resided sought judicial guidance, surgery had become necessary for the tube to be replaced. The court refused to order this surgery, claiming that the burdens of the procedure would outweigh its benefits for her. The court's benefit-burden analysis was problematic, to say the least. Although the opinion expresses concern about the procedure's 20 percent mortality risk (due to the patient's advanced age), it omits any mention of the 100 percent mortality risk of nonfeeding. The court also predicted that if the tube were reinserted, the patient would simply pull it out again. Finally, the court characterized Hier's actions as a "plea for privacy and personal dignity by a ninety-two-year-old person who is seriously ill and for whom life has little left to offer" (464 N.E.2d at 965).

The shortcomings in this case resemble those in *Spring*. The *Hier* court failed to examine what life *did* have to offer this patient. Did she obtain enjoyment from any activities and interactions, or was she uncomfortable and withdrawn from the world? (She reportedly believed she was the queen of England—not a bad sort of existence, in my opinion! [Annas, 1984, p. 23]) The court also failed to consider how the patient would experience nontreatment—how this conscious patient would experience death from dehydration and malnutrition. Here again, we see a court focusing on an image of a competent patient concerned with privacy and dignity, rather than on the patient herself. There is no realization that the act of pulling out the tube could reflect a very different mental state in this patient, such as mild irritation at the apparatus or staff, or a wish for attention. (She had recently been transferred to the nursing home and perhaps was feeling lonely and isolated.) Concern for privacy and dignity instead was attributed to a demented patient who probably was unaware of and unconcerned with these matters. The dangers of this approach also are revealed in *Hier*, for the affidavit of one of the two physicians testifying against the surgery stated that he thought she had consumed "enough" scarce health care resources in her lifetime, and no more should be expended on her (Annas, 1984). The court omitted this as an explicit reason for its decision, yet it did stress that two of the three physicians testifying were against the surgery. (In the end, Hier was treated; her legal representative went back to the trial court, produced additional medical testimony that the surgery would benefit her, and the surgery was ordered. The appellate decision still stands as a precedent to guide future cases, however.)

These two cases demonstrate some of the problems created by the current legal approach and its search to determine what incompetent patients would want if they were competent. The failure to direct attention to the patient's current welfare allows troubling trade-offs between patients' interests and the interests of others. It is crucial to keep social judgments on what constitutes dignified treatment for demented patients from overriding such patients' clear and demonstrable interests in receiving treatment. It is also crucial to prevent such judgments from masking less altruistic concerns, such as the emotional and monetary burdens these patients' lives impose on their families and the broader society. At times, it may be appropriate to consider these burdens, but they ought not be protectively cloaked in the guise of the patients' well-being or privacy and dignity.

THE NEED FOR CONSENSUAL STANDARDS

Precedent autonomy is not the solution to our current dilemmas regarding life-sustaining treatment for incompetent patients. Besides its inherent moral problems, its practical scope is likely to remain small. It is rare to encounter a true exercise of precedent autonomy involving an incompetent patient's medical treatment. Few people make advance directives, and those who do usually speak with substantial imprecision. Although the numbers might increase with education and other policy efforts, I believe that many and perhaps most persons will continue, consciously or inadvertently, to leave life-and-death matters unattended. Indeed, it is estimated that only one-third of Americans have property wills when they die (Malcolm, 1990).

We need default rules to govern the numerous cases in which incompetent patients have failed to exercise precedent autonomy. Moreover, we need rules setting forth the acceptable boundaries of precedent autonomy and proxy decision-making. Just as there are legal limits on the range of treatment choices parents may make for their children, so should there be limits on the range of choices competent persons have concerning their future treatment and the choices available to proxy decision-makers in general. In short, we as a society must take a moral and legal stand on which categories of incompetent patients must be treated and which may have treatment forgone.

The task, admittedly, is formidable, and one that we have assiduously sought to avoid. Indeed, the customary focus on autonomy to answer these questions has in part been an evasive maneuver. Generating consensual standards on treatment requires judgments on quality of life. Decisions must be made on which patients obtain a significant enough benefit from treatment and continued life to obligate others to maintain that life. Such decisions are difficult, unsettling, and understandably shunned. But I believe that they are the best means both of protecting the interests of incompetent patients and of avoiding inappropriate overtreatment of such patients.

Recent commentators have ably defended quality-of-life judgments from the customary charges of immorality and abuse. Buchanan and Brock noted that treatment standards focused on patient well-being must incorporate quality-of-life determinations (Buchanan and Brock, 1986, p. 73). For example, a decision to forgo ICU care that could provide a terminally ill incompetent patient with a few weeks of extended life entailing constant discomfort is a decision that the patient's quality of life in that state is too burdensome to mandate treatment. Similarly, a decision to forgo dialysis for a persistently vegetative patient involves a judgment that the patient's quality of life is insufficient to make continued life a benefit to that patient. The crucial requirement is that such evaluations ask what value life holds for the individual incompetent patient. The evaluations must be *intra*personal, directed at determining how a specific patient experiences life. Such evaluations are to be distinguished from morally inappropriate social-worth evaluations, which would base treatment on an individual's ability to contribute to society (Buchanan and Brock, 1986).

We must also recognize that quality-of-life judgments have not been, and probably cannot be, avoided in treatment decision-making (Rhoden, 1985). It is better to make them openly, with an explicit and systematic focus on the individual patient's contemporaneous interests, than to cloak them in the guise of autonomy, or what the patient "would want" if competent. Conspicuous and openly performed quality-of-life assessments also can guard against the possibility of subordinating the patient's interests to the concerns of others, such as emotionally distressed family members or financially strapped health care institutions.

In sum, we need to devote our efforts to forging consensual treatment standards for incompetent patients. Legal and ethical debate should center on deciding what levels of awareness and benefit give incompetent patients a significant enough interest in life to require others to provide continued medical treatment. The present interest in advance directives, as well as numerous public surveys and other studies, reveals emerging agreement that life-sustaining medical technology is inappropriate in certain circumstances. Now the boundaries must be further refined and more precise normative standards formulated (Dresser, 1988). It is an intimidating and troubling project. Yet I believe that undertaking it will lead to a more honest appraisal of the genuine competing interests at stake in these difficult cases.

REFERENCES

Annas, G. (1984). The case of Mary Hier: when substituted judgment becomes sleight of hand. *Hastings Center Report, 14*(4):23–25.

Arras, J. (1984). Toward an ethics of ambiguity. *Hastings Center Report, 14*(2):30–31.

Barber v. Superior Court (1983). 147 Cal. App.3d 1006, 195 Cal. Rptr. 484.

Brophy v. New England Sinai Hospital (1986). 398 Mass. 417, 497 N.E.2d 626.

Buchanan, A. (1988). Advance directives and the personal identity problem. *Philosophy and Public Affairs, 17*:277–302.

Buchanan, A., and Brock, D.W. (1986). Deciding for others. *Milbank Quarterly, 64*(Supplement 2):17–94.

Cruzan v. Harmon (1989). 760 S.W.2d 408 (Mo. 1988), *certiorari granted,* 109 S.CT. 3240 (#88-1503).

Dennett, D. (1987). *The Intentional Stance.* Cambridge: MIT Press.

Dresser, R. (1988). Life, death, and incompetent patients: conceptual infirmities and hidden values in the law. *Arizona Law Review, 28*(3):388–405.

Dresser, R. (1990). Relitigating life and death. *Ohio State Law Journal, 51*:425–437.

Dresser, R., and Robertson, J. (1989). Quality of life and non-treatment decisions for incompetent patients: a critique of the orthodox approach. *Law, Medicine and Health Care, 17*(3):234–244.

Dworkin, R. (1986). Autonomy and the demented self. *Milbank Quarterly, 64*(Supplement 2):4–16.

Ellman, I.M. (1990). Can others exercise an incapacitated patient's right to die? *Hastings Center Report, 20*(1):47–50.

Evans v. Bellevue Hospital (1987). *New York Law Journal* (July 28):11.

Howell, M. (1984). Caretakers' views on responsibilities for the care of the demented elderly. *Journal of the American Geriatrics Society, 32*(9):657–660.

In re Conroy (1985). 98 N.J. 321, 486 A.2d 1209.

In re Hier (1984). 18 Mass. App. 200, 464 N.E.2d 959; *appeal denied* (1984), 392 Mass. 1102, 465 N.E.2d 261.

In re Jobes (1987). 108 N.J. 394, 529 A.2d 434.

In re Quinlan (1976). 70 N.J. 10, 355 A.2d 647.

In re Spring (1980). 380 Mass. 629, 405 N.E.2d 115.

In re Westchester County Medical Center (1988). 72 N.Y.2d 517, 531 N.E.2d 607.

Malcolm, A. (1990). Two right-to-die groups merging for unified voice. *New York Times* (April 4):A12.

Nagel, T. (1986). *The View from Nowhere.* New York: Oxford University Press.

President's Commission for the Study of Ethical Problems in Medicine and Biomedical and Behavioral Research (1983). *Deciding to Forgo Life-Sustaining Treatment.* Washington, D.C.: U.S. Government Printing Office.

Rhoden, N.K. (1985). Treatment dilemmas for imperiled newborns: why quality of life counts. *Southern California Law Review, 58*:1283–1347.

Rhoden, N.K. (1988). Litigating life and death. *Harvard Law Review, 102*: 375–446.

Rhoden, N.K. (1990). The limits of legal objectivity. *North Carolina Law Review, 68*:845–865.

Weir, R. (1989). *Abating Treatment with Critically Ill Patients.* New York: Oxford University Press.

7

A CRITICAL VIEW OF ETHICAL DILEMMAS IN DEMENTIA

Harry R. Moody

I may venture to affirm that we are nothing but a bundle or collection of different sensations, which succeed each other with an inconceivable rapidity, and are in perpetual flux and movement.

—David Hume, *Treatise on Human Nature*

You have to begin to lose your memory, if only in bits and pieces, to realize that memory is what makes our lives. Life without memory is no life at all. . . . Our memory is our coherence, our reason, our feeling, even our action. Without it, we are nothing. . . . I can only wait for the final amnesia, the one that can erase an entire life, as it did my mother's.

—Luis Buñuel

THE PHENOMENOLOGY OF DEMENTIA

In his book on the phenomenology of illness, James Buchanan (1989) has a piercing chapter on the experience of Alzheimer's disease. He recounts the story of "Murray Wasserman," a 57-year-old man stricken with early-onset Alzheimer's. As the disease progresses, Murray's memory loss and confusion become progressively worse. Yet the terror of the situation is that this patient still recognizes what is happening and foresees what lies in the future. This awareness of vulnerability casts its shadow over all his relationships and finally compromises what the patient takes to be his own dignity.

The contemporary literature on bioethics too quickly tends to conflate the ideals of "dignity" and "autonomy." Ethical theory assures us that we honor a patient's dignity by respecting that patient's autonomy to make decisions. The moment of decision tends to become the focus of ethical deliberation, while background elements of the situation, including human relationships, are lost from sight.

Yet this way of thinking about the problem may be what misleads us. We cannot grasp the dilemmas of dementia in a case study or a snapshot at a single moment of time. It is the whole history of the disease, of the patient, of relationships, which is crucial. In the slow deterioration of Alzheimer's disease the erosion of real autonomy takes place long before major decisions come into question.

The loss experienced by the patient is not a matter of rationality or even self-determination. It is shame, a loss of dignity in the eyes of others, a loss compounded by the fact that others adapt to the situation, become accustomed to the patient's incompetence, and finally come to consider the patient less than a person. The dementia sufferer resembles Gregor Samsa, the hero of Kafka's story "The Metamorphosis," who awoke one morning to discover that he had become changed into a huge insect. Kafka proceeds to give us all the details of how Samsa's family and associates reacted to the event: first with horror, then gradual adaptation. So too, the dementia victim takes on the feature of an infrahuman animal, a pet, who lives among human beings but no longer shares their world. This is the horror Kafka evokes for us.

Yet Kafka's story is inadequate too, and for the same reason that the bioethics literature fails us in trying to grasp dementia. In "The Metamorphosis" the transition to the subhuman state is abrupt; it literally happens overnight. So too, in the literature of bioethics we have abrupt encounters with patients. In case studies, patients are typically seen at a single moment in time. We encounter patients who have already arrived at their demented state. But by the time they are of interest for ethical analysis, they have lost mental capacity, and so they become a "problem" for medical or family decision-makers. Who will be the surrogate? How much to take account of previous intentions expressed by the patient? What about fluctuating capacity?

All are difficult questions, yet somehow the questions miss the crucial fact about dementia, which is that we call it an "illness" yet it is an illness of a very peculiar kind. The situation resembles the film *The Invasion of the Body Snatchers*, where alien invaders take over the bodies of ordinary people who continue to resemble their previous selves. Like the relatives of those who are possessed by the body snatchers, relatives of dementia victims can deceive themselves for a time into thinking that things are normal. Pretending that things are still normal is not just denial; it is a way of grasping at hope and dignity, of holding the nightmare at bay, as disorder unfolds in the midst of ordinary human relationships, disrupting them and preserving them at the same time.

"Insidious onset" is the diagnostic label used by neurologists to characterize the disease. The lived reality is something else again. "Your husband looks so healthy" is the comment typically made by friends who visit someone caring for a person in the early stages of dementia. The progress of the disorder is insidious, the possibilities for denial endless. In later stages, denial is no longer possible. Different problems arise, including, finally, the classic bioethical dilemmas—paternalistic intervention, termination of treatment, equity in bearing the burdens of caregiving (Hermann, 1984; Cassel and Goldstein, 1988).

Then, in the final stages of the disease, we come back to the question of how we are to understand the suffering of the patient or the caregiver. What do we say about the aged mother who no longer recognizes her own son? Is the patient "no longer there," despite the illusion, the replica, that persists like an afterimage before our eyes? Can we represent to ourselves what the loss of the self finally means? Do we have a literature adequate to the horror of dementia? Perhaps we will find that literature only in the theater of the absurd, in the fragments of "stream of consciousness" fiction, in the word salad of *Finnegans Wake*. But even if we guard against simplistic metaphors, in the end we need some means of making sense of the suffering and giving guidance for the ethical decisions that must be made.

DEMENTIA AND THE DOMINANT MODEL IN BIOETHICS

Ethicists today make use of rational principles to give guidance in normative ethics—for example, by appealing to principles of beneficence, autonomy, and justice, ideals that can properly be described as the "big three" of contemporary biomedical ethics (President's Commission for the Study of Ethical Problems in Medicine, 1983). These foundational principles are found enshrined whenever we come upon what one might call "consensus" documents giving ethical guidance to clinicians and policymakers, and their appeal is understandable. But here I want to take a different approach and look instead at the "dark side" of these principles. Let me begin with beneficence.

THE TEMPTATIONS OF BENEFICENCE

Every year we are accustomed to seeing a newspaper story about someone, typically a spouse or adult child, who deals with a demented relative by means of beneficent euthanasia—that is, killing people "for their own good." In these cases the killer makes no attempt to flee but explains the action by saying that the dementia victim was "better off dead" or perhaps was "already dead" or "no longer human," even a "vegetable."

Now to speak of patients this way is to employ dangerous language. We should recall that in *The Invasion of the Body Snatchers* the psychological hurdle for the humans was in learning to kill "pod people" who had "taken over" human beings. Once it is possible to say that they are not human at all but only "impostors," then killing becomes easier. In the same way, once we can convince ourselves that end-stage Alzheimer's patients are "no longer there" or are less than fully human, then it becomes easier to kill them.

The danger of beneficence is that there are powerful attractions to killing people, particularly to overburdened caregivers who begin to think of the patient as already dead. In the words of one caregiver: "It's like a funeral that never ends." Again: "Sometimes I wish he would die so that it would be over. It seems as if he is dying a bit at a time, day after day. When something new happens I think I can't stand it" (Mace and Rabins, 1983, p. 164).

This is just the level of desperation which has prompted some of the highly publicized incidents of "mercy killing." Apart from the legal liability for homicide, there are moral issues that arise in similar cases where outright killing is not the issue—for example, where the patient is "allowed to die." The justification for either active or passive euthanasia in these instances illustrates the troubling dilemmas associated with dementia.

Caregiver burden complicates a realistic determination of the patient's best interest. Dementing illness constitutes a tremendous emotional burden on a family. In assessing the stress on caregivers, we cannot afford to count on unremitting love or tolerance. That would be a standard of saintliness, not of ordinary human virtue. This is obviously not the standard by which it is easy to contemplate "beneficent euthanasia" or perhaps even to think of family members as surrogate decision-makers.

An unlimited principle of beneficence is dangerous when applied to dementia precisely because an appeal to the principle of autonomy becomes less and less plausible as a counterweight. With no barrier from autonomy, an appeal to beneficence may persuade us that euthanasia is the best course for the patient. But if a patient "looks" normal, it may require a high degree of "psychological distancing" for us to overcome the normal moral repugnance at killing, or allowing to die, as with the "pod people." We are dealing, after all, with someone who "looks like us." Overcoming that distance is possible, but perhaps at the cost of diminishing our moral sensibilities.

For these reasons, I believe it is crucial to uphold the line that forbids direct killing—active euthanasia—and to maintain a considerable degree of scrutiny over medical decisions at the end of life with demented patients. Societal scrutiny need not insist on sanctity of life as an absolute principle. But it should act from a principle of prudence in not permitting irrevocable acts to be done when intolerable pressures are likely to arise, as they do in the care of dementia patients.

It is just here that we can grasp the danger of thinking about the ethics of dementia in terms of the analogy of animal rights or any view that makes dementia patients into something less than human (Brock, 1988). The argument is that patients in end-stage dementia are hardly any longer "persons." It has been suggested that, like a fetus, they have more in common with higher animals than with rational adult human beings.

But this analogy is bound to be disturbing to devoted caregivers, and for good reason. The animal-rights model is mistaken because "animal rights" seems to leave open the prospect that individual organisms can be directly killed to satisfy more compelling human needs, just as we kill animals for food. Once killing is accepted with end-stage dementia patients, if the animal-rights analogy is accepted, then there is nothing to prevent us from extending the practice to other subrational organisms: neonates, the severely retarded, or others.

In sounding this note of caution and invoking a "slippery slope" argument, we need not go to the opposite extreme. It is reasonable for families, and for society as a whole, to debate openly just what kind of treatment is appropriate for a future in which vast numbers of end-stage Alzheimer's patients will populate our nursing homes and will command the resources from families and government (Office of Technology Assessment, 1987). Drawing a line here will not be easy. But if we decide to be less than heroic with end-stage demented patients, we should do so not because we tell ourselves that these patients are no more than animals but rather because we as a society make a "tragic choice" in the same way that we do in ordering soldiers into battle, foreseeing loss of life but not directly intending it (Calabresi and Bobbitt, 1974).

ILLUSIONS OF AUTONOMY

In thinking about the ethics of dementia, it is critical to understand why it is not autonomy but dignity or self-respect that should be the primary value. A crucial part of one's self-respect is respect in the eyes of others, and this need has deeper roots than rationality or self-determination. Respect is related to shame. Both are inseparable from one's identity and visibility in a social order.

Yet the prevailing outlook in bioethics, along with modern culture as a whole, tends to overlook ideals such as honor or dignity at the same time as prizing individual autonomy as an imperative of liberal society. Autonomy is construed as the essential bedrock of "respect for persons," a constituent element of personhood itself, and thus it becomes the foundation for contemporary bioethics.

A major ethical imperative that follows from this supremacy of autonomy can be found in the current enthusiasm for advance directives, both the living will and the durable power of attorney for health affairs. Now to argue against advance directives is a bit like arguing against peace treaties to end conflict among nations. After all, who can be against peace? But this way of posing the question is itself mistaken. The issue is not whether treaties are desirable, but rather what might be conditions that make a formal, legal agreement at all possible. After all, there are treaties that are not merely useless but actually misleading and damaging. Still other treaties serve only to ratify the weakening of rights of weaker parties. Finally, there is the fact that when the treaty is most needed—that is, to stop the battle—it may, as a practical matter, be least available.

All these problems apply in the case of advance directives for dementia. Advance directives can be deceptive. They can actually weaken rights we already have, and they are often unusable at just the time when they are most needed. As legal instruments, advance directives always remain subject to the power of the state. There are more than a few cases where legislatures proceed to write into law a prohibition that removes rights that citizens already have under common law—the right, for instance, to refuse artificial hydration and nutrition. It is not obvious that advance directives that ratify the weakening of rights represent any sort of progress.

Further, there are problems of justice in sorting out the competing claims of family members, in addressing professional or institutional fears, and in making claims when "too much" treatment is demanded, such as when doctors agree that treatment is "futile" but surrogates demand it anyway. Regardless of what a durable power of attorney may say, it is simply an illusion to imagine that health care institutions will feel relieved of their obligation to consult with all involved family members in a termination-of-treatment decision, especially if one troublesome family member threatens lawsuit.

Then too, as a practical matter, advance directives are most effective in helping patients to refuse treatment, but not to secure treatment. The reasons are obvious. Refusing treatment is simply not parallel with the expense of demanding treatment. At some point the autonomy claims embodied in advanced directives run up against resource constraints and counterclaims of distributive justice.

Finally, we have the clinical reality of dementia itself. Diagnosis is difficult, denial is pervasive, and the prognosis or staging of the disease is often uncertain in its timing. Here, as elsewhere in human affairs, timing is everything. By the time a patient and family have received a diagnosis and come to accept the reality, it may be too late to engage in planning for incapacity. Just as many people die without making a will, so remarkably few will have advance directives to help chart the course of their treatment.

All this does not mean that advance directives are useless, any more than peace treaties are useless in international affairs. But the heart of the matter is not to be found in the legal instrument as much as in the process of communication and negotiation which leads up to the result. Every stage of dementia involves renegotiating goals, expectations, rights, and obligations. There will never be a legal instrument or a simple paper process that gives us an escape from this demanding process of communication among parties to a decision. Advance directives in dementia have their uses—for example, to facilitate wider communication among interested parties. But it is a dangerous illusion to imagine that they can somehow dispense with the serious and ongoing challenge of communication and negotiation.

THE AMBIGUITIES OF JUSTICE

Let me turn finally to justice. Most discussions of distributive justice in bioethics are based on a macromodel of justice. They begin with considerations about society as a whole with the national government as the preferred agency for deciding on allocation of resources. But this view is incomplete because many of the most difficult problems of distributive justice arise at other levels of social life—for example, in reconciling competing claims among family members. The dilemmas of distributive justice are unavoidable in the case of the dependent elderly, where the bulk of hands-on care is provided by families.

An analysis of justice at the level of the family is likely to yield conflicting imperatives because it is impossible to disentangle abstract claims or duties from the concrete historical relationships of individuals. Does the sole daughter or son who has been subjected to lifelong neglect, or worse, from a parent now suddenly find an obligation to provide care for that failing parent? What happens if caregiving demands reach heroic proportions? At the level of society as a whole, large numbers can smooth over or average out burdens—for example, by taxation or by monetizing exchanges. But small groups, like the family, depend on discontinuous acts by individuals. Even if we were to agree on equal sharing of the caregiving burden by siblings, contingencies such as geographic proximity, gender roles, or interpersonal relationships conspire to make the burdens unequal, and often unfair, in practice.

Moreover, there are certain kinds of help which only families can give precisely because of the power of lifelong relationships. It is a deep illusion to imagine that government can somehow substitute for that help. No conceivable army of social workers can substitute for the visit of a loving child who cares for an aged parent in the hour of need. No one else will have the kind of shared, historical knowledge that belongs to the particular relationship between parent and child. Filial obligation arises from the fact that a son or daughter is the only one who can provide a certain help that is needed. The duty is intensely particular, not general, and it needs an ethics of particularity to make it intelligible.

Concrete relationships, in other words, are crucial. To say this is not to romanticize relationships or to imagine that relationships as such solve all problems of justice. The task of wisdom is to see caregiving for the aged as a "shared function" between the family and formal organizations. In Plato's phrase, justice demands giving each function its due. But the reality of relationship and the primacy of respect for persons rooted in concrete experience means that justice must be differentiated in its different spheres (Walzer, 1983).

TOWARD A COMMUNICATIVE ETHICS

If prevailing principles and approaches of bioethics are not adequate to the phenomenological reality of dementia, then where shall we turn for an analytic approach to the ethical dilemmas posed by the disorder? I want to sketch out one such approach derived from critical theory as elaborated by Habermas (1990). The broad conclusion here is that in place of an abstract ethics of rules or principles, we need a communicative ethics grounded in practice and in lived experience.

PRIMACY OF COMMUNICATION

The first implication of communicative ethics is the primacy of communication both on the clinical level and throughout the wider society. This point has implications for current legal debates about informed consent. In clinical decision-making, the primacy of communication suggests that we reject the standards of *both* the best-interest and substituted judgment insofar as they purport to be final or definitive principles for deciding on behalf of incompetent patients (Dresser, 1990). Abstract principles like autonomy and beneficence are secondary to the social process of communication itself.

Specifically, I would argue that we abandon the belief that advance directives can be an adequate means of safeguarding the autonomy of a prior "intact self" in order to bind the future demented self. We should also abandon the idea that caregivers should make discretionary decisions based on a standard of beneficence toward the demented individual. Both autonomy and beneficence revolve around claims of individuals. In place of that focus on individuals, we should put the attention on the *social structure* in which communication takes place. Instead of the fiction of autonomy or the temptations of beneficence, we should recognize that caregiving for Alzheimer's disease entails irreducible questions of social justice and the social meaning of dementia.

I add that this line of criticism is not a wholesale argument against using advance directives for those with dementia, particularly now that the Supreme Court's *Cruzan* decision makes it more necessary, at least in some jurisdictions, to obtain "clear and convincing evidence" of a patient's prior treatment preference. But this legal standard is likely to prove unrealistic in practice, as ethicists have warned.

Whatever principles prevail on the legal level, we need an ethical standard and a process of decision for those caring for persons with dementia. Advance directives have a place in that process, but we need to think about advance planning in a different way. We should think of advance directives as occasions for communication, not as a means of definitively settling treatment decisions. For the patient whose mental competence is irrevocably lost, advance directives offer valuable pieces of evidence about a patient's intentions. But, like all evidence, they are subject to interpretation, qualification, and negotiation as circumstances change.

We should not think of advance directives as quasi-contractual instruments. If a living will, for example, is thought of as a substitute for conversation between doctor and patient, then it becomes a dangerous illusion. On the contrary, the chief virtue of encouraging dementia patients and their families to undertake advance directives may be that the very act of writing the living will or making the power of attorney provides an occasion for getting all concerned parties—patient, family members, health care professionals—to talk to one another about treatment decisions. Ambivalence and confusion may remain, but the activity of communication fulfills its purpose.

NEGOTIATION

Many of the dilemmas of autonomy in geriatric ethics are better conceived in terms of "negotiated consent" rather than informed consent (Moody, 1988). But what is "negotiation" and does it really offer a way out of conflict? In fact, getting the parties together to communicate may lead to conflict rather than immediate consensus. In the real world of decision-making, different, and sometimes opposing, interests are at stake. To acknowledge that point is another way of talking about politics at the microscale in families and clinical settings. The essence of politics at any scale involves the reconciliation of competing interests: in short, who gets what, when, and how, as Lasswell put it (Lasswell, 1958). We should recognize political bargaining and negotiation as indispensable and legitimate elements in ethical decision-making.

To stress the importance of politics is not necessarily to reject altogether methods of promoting individual autonomy, such as advance directives. In fact, a more forthright acknowledgment of the politics of practice may be crucial if advance directives are to be anything more than an exercise in futility. When a proxy or surrogate is granted legal authority to make decisions, the authority to refuse treatment, as a practical matter, is never going to be as absolute as the authority of the competent patient him- or herself, whatever ethical theory may suggest. In practice, proxy decision-makers need all the help they can get if they are to be empowered to act de facto on behalf of demented patients, whatever the law prescribes. Helping proxies means recognizing the political realities they must cope with in the clinical setting.

While empowering proxy decision-makers, we need also to recognize that there are other interested parties with a legitimate stake in the outcome, including, for example, family members, professional caregivers, and health care institutions. These different parties may have opposing views about what to do. To speak of these as "legitimate stakeholders" is not to put them all at the same level. It is simply to recognize that these parties must have their views recognized and somehow taken into account. The criteria for legitimacy will vary and are themselves subject to debate. But then, that is the whole point of insisting that negotiation is the appropriate metaphor for the micropolitics of clinical decision-making. It is from the model of politics and negotiation, not from law or juridical principles, that we should seek guidance in trying to find a resolution to the dilemmas at hand.

MORAL AMBIGUITY

It is vital to acknowledge the "ethics of ambiguity" in dementia (Arras, 1984). Some of the ambiguities are empirical or diagnostic. The insidious onset of the disorder poses difficult questions—for example, deciding whether a given patient has a specific dementing illness, predicting the timing and probable course of the disease, separating out secondary psychiatric reactions from the primary process of the disease. These empirical medical questions are critical in terms of thinking about the meaning of the disease both for the patient and for the family.

Closely related to diagnostic ambiguity is the question of whether we should think of Alzheimer's disease as a "terminal" illness. In political terms, the concept of "terminality" legitimates acts that foreseeably result in the patient's death. There is no clear or simple way to separate the empirical ambiguities about the trajectory of the disease from the moral ambiguities about our response to it.

A further point about moral ambiguity arises from the uncertain cognitive status of the dementia patient over the course of the disease. An ethics of principles is poorly suited to deal with the changing moral status of the demented. Most legal and ethical thinking in bioethics is dominated by the idea of duties toward persons—that is, moral agents capable of responsibility. Even a patient completely unconscious retains these rights of personhood. What then is the moral status of the demented? What happens when a disease, like Alzheimer's, erodes the foundations of moral agency and personality? The phenomenon of dementia necessarily raises profound questions about personal identity and the meaning of the self.

FAMILY DECISION-MAKING

An important line of thought recently has moved to acknowledge explicitly the authority of the family as the primary decision-maker in cases where the patient has become incompetent (Rhoden, 1988). Of course the family has always functioned in this surrogate role, in informal ways and in varying degrees. But shifting responsibility in a definitive or principled way to families may have some unwelcome consequences. For example, families sometimes act out of guilt or despair in demanding overtreatment for end-stage Alzheimer's patients. We hear families say *"Do everything* for my mother"—even if the patient is 90 years old and severely demented and has no reasonable hope of recovery.

So the question emerges: What status should we give to "family consent"? There are reasons for not answering this question in too definitive a fashion. Indeed, there are some advantages to insisting on the moral ambiguity of the situation and refusing to set up clear principles for decision-making. Any theory of surrogate decision-making through the family must come to grips with the reality of guilt. It is one thing to solicit the family's views in a consultative fashion through negotiation. It is something quite different to convert the family into a presumptive surrogate as a matter of principle. Again, I argue that we should reject this appeal to principle in favor of an ethic of ambiguity. The appropriate response to moral ambiguity is the response of communication.

CULTURE AND MEANING

We need to raise questions about what it means for dementia to be understood as a "disease." In putting the matter this way, I do not mean to question the organic etiology of the disorder but rather to call into question the way in which the medicalization of Alzheimer's disease entails some serious losses for patients and their families. In Alzheimer's, the same behavior once described as "senility" is now categorized and labeled as a disease. Yet the disorder remains incurable. What was once a matter for families to cope with as best they could now becomes identified as a problem demanding "professional" intervention. Yet professional intervention comes at a cost, both in money and in more subtle ways. Habermas, for example, spoke of the "colonization of the life-world" by which instrumental categories of professional ideology come to dominate all forms of human experience. We see the consequences of this professional ideology in the case of the medical model of dementia.

The medical model constitutes a specific mode of interpreting human experience, including the experience of illness. The medical model adopts an instrumental, rather than a hermeneutic, view of experience. Specifically, the medical model entails a causal-reductive approach that excludes dimensions of meaning, above all the meaning of suffering.

The loss of meaning for Alzheimer's disease has some very specific ethical consequences. Because the medical model can offer little hope of cure, it is not surprising that care for the demented, like the handicapped, remains a backwater bypassed by the technological orientation of professional health care. Doctors aren't often interested in incurable disorders with difficult behavioral consequences. But then, do we really want the management of dementia to be taken over by a medical model? The implications of wholesale medicalization are likely to be professional domination, soaring costs, and, not least, deep dilemmas of allocating available services. Perhaps a social rather than a medical model for care of the demented will prove not only less expensive but more humane as well, as the hospice experience has suggested in the case of terminal illness.

There is a further disturbing implication of the medical model and the loss of meaning in dementia. In modern societies, dominated by the instrumental logic of professional ideology, patients who are in the end stages of dementia must appear as beings less than fully human. The next step, according to the logic of instrumental efficiency, would be to discount their right to existence—since a demented existence is meaningless. A pure "best-interest" standard of surrogate decision-making might logically acquiesce in deliberately ending the lives of the demented, since those lives have already lost all meaning. How we respond to this prospect will depend on whether we can envisage dementia in a wider societal context of meaning, which alone can address the vexing issues raised here (Cole and Gadow, 1986).

THE SOCIETAL DIMENSION

In the last decade Alzheimer's disease has moved, in the famous phrase of sociologist C. Wright Mills, from a private sorrow to being understood as a public problem. This accomplishment was made possible by vigorous advocacy on the part of the Alzeimer's disease movement, which made Alzheimer's more visible in the public arena. For good or ill, dementia has become understood as a disease and has thus entered into the political dimension by which society copes with medical problems. It is part of my argument to insist that this political dimension—from negotiation to advocacy—is indispensable to understanding what is at stake in the ethical dilemmas of dementia. Instead of the value-neutral, depoliticized instrumental logic of the "medical model," we need to understand how both the disease and clinical intervention are located within a wider societal discourse. This requires in turn a reappraisal of the cognitive interests that shape our understanding.

What made possible the success of the Alzheimer's disease movement was a very specific social experience—namely, the organization of mutual self-help groups of caregivers for Alzheimer's victims. As in other forms of the self-help movement, caregivers came together in regular, informal meetings and shared their most private and painful experiences with one another. These mutual support groups proved to be successful vehicles for promoting what Habermas would call "communicative competence." Where caregivers once experienced private rage or despair, when they came together they discovered a form of mutual experience which overcame individual isolation.

This was not an accidental discovery but a socially structured process. As Gubrium documented, members of caregiver support groups actually learned a new language in which to redescribe their subjective experience. Their achievement of a communicative breakthrough at the small scale proved essential to subsequent success at communicating to the larger society what is at stake in Alzheimer's disease and what kind of care and treatment is needed (Gubrium, 1988).

This same historical process is recapitulated, again and again, among families who come to experience Alzheimer's disease for the first time. From the standpoint of critical theory, this process expresses an emancipatory interest, a demand for liberation. The movement constitutes a transition away from a passive, instrumentalized mode of thinking—

for example, "Is there a cure for what's wrong with my husband?"—to higher levels of communicative competence involving both a hermeneutic or interpretive mode and ultimately a level of empowerment. Empowerment means overcoming the feeling of isolation and helplessness which comes with an incurable disease. The paradox is that empowerment and vulnerability go together. By asking questions about the meaning of suffering, individuals in the support group come to experience their suffering in a different way. Empowerment does not mean finding a cure but rather taking power over our experience. Instead of feelings of chaos or unfairness ("Why me?"), empowerment means recovering dignity, hope, and a sense of meaning—in short, a reason to go on living in the midst of tragedy.

Communicative ethics, derived from critical theory, would insist that we look at the ethical dilemmas of dementia in terms of a wider cognitive interest than those we ordinarily take into account in bioethics or public policy. It would challenge the discourse of individual autonomy and professional ideology and instead reassert the primacy of interpretation and empowerment as categories for ethical analysis. Communicative ethics, in sum, offers a powerful alternative to the ethics of rules and principles so pervasive in contemporary thinking about ethical issues. For geriatric ethics, and specifically for the ethical dilemmas of dementia, we need a wider perspective that acknowledges moral ambiguity, raises questions about the meaning of disease, and, above all, insists on the primacy of communication (Moody, in press).

There will continue to be a fundamental power and centrality for ethics in the "big three" principles of autonomy, beneficence, and justice. By criticizing the temptations, illusions, and ambiguities involved in those principles, my intention has been to show why an alternative framework—communicative ethics—can remedy some of the weaknesses of prevailing methods of bioethics. But any perspective, communicative or not, will unavoidably fail to capture the full phenomenological reality of what it means to be sick, to be dying, to be demented. Much as we need to hear alternative voices in the theoretical debate of bioethics, even more so do we need to hear the voice of all the victims and caregivers who cope with the moral dilemmas of dementia in their daily lives.

REFERENCES

Arras, J. (1984). Toward an ethic of ambiguity. *Hastings Center Report*, *14*(2):25–33.

Brock, D.W. (1988). Justice and the severely demented elderly. *Journal of Medicine and Philosophy*, *13*:73–99.

Buchanan, J.H. (1989). *Patient Encounters: The Experience of Disease*. Charlottesville, Va.: University Press of Virginia.

Calabresi, G., and Bobbitt, P. (1974). *Tragic Choices*. New York: W.W. Norton.

Cassel, C.K., and Goldstein, M.K. (1988). Ethical considerations. In L. Jarvik, ed., *Treatments for the Alzheimer's Patient: The Long Haul*, pp. 80–95. New York: Springer Publishing Co.

Cole, T., and Gadow, S., eds. (1986). *What Does It Mean to Grow Old? Views from the Humanities*. Durham, N.C.: Duke University Press.

Dresser, R. (1990). Relitigating life and death. *Ohio State Law Journal*, *51*:425–437.

Gubrium, J. (1988). *Oldtimers and Alzheimer's: The Social Construction of Senility*. Westport, Conn.: Greenwood Press.

Habermas, J. (1990). *Moral Consciousness and Communicative Action*, translated by Christian Lenhardt and Shierry Weber Nicholsen, Cambridge: MIT Press.

Hermann, H.T. (1984). Ethical dilemmas intrinsic to the care of the elderly demented patient. *Journal of the American Geriatric Society*, *32*(9):655–656.

Lasswell, H. (1958). *Politics: Who Gets What, When, How*. New York: World Publishing Co.

Mace, N.L., and Rabins, P.V. (1983). *The 36-Hour Day*. Baltimore, Md.: Johns Hopkins University Press.

Moody, H.R. (1988). From informed consent to negotiated consent. *Gerontologist*, *28*(Supplement):76–70.

Moody, H.R. (In press). *Ethics and Aging*. Baltimore, Md.: Johns Hopkins University Press.

Office of Technology Assessment, Congress of the United States. (1987). *Losing a Million Minds: Confronting the Tragedy of Alzheimer's Disease and Other Dementias*. Washington, D.C.: U.S. Government Printing Office.

President's Commission for the Study of Ethical Problems in Medicine. (1983). *Securing Access to Health Care*. Washington, D.C.: U.S. Government Printing Office.

Rhoden, N.K. (1988). Litigating life and death. *Harvard Law Review*, *102*:375–446.

Walzer, M. (1983). *Spheres of Justice*. New York: Basic Books.

8

MERCY KILLING OF ELDERLY PEOPLE WITH DEMENTIA: A COUNTERPROPOSAL

David C. Thomasma

Several years ago Mrs. Janet Adkins of Oregon, diagnosed as having Alzheimer's disease, requested Dr. Jack Kevorkian of Michigan to assist her suicide. After assuring himself that she was a mentally competent person, he did so. She had read of his invention, an intravenous device that dripped deadly chemicals into one's veins. As a member of the Hemlock Society, Mrs. Adkins believed that individuals should have the right to die with dignity. Dr. Kevorkian's device permits the individual to push a button to inaugurate a chemical death. It is foolproof. There can be no botched suicide attempt. So Mrs. Adkins dispatched herself with his help in a van in a Michigan park. Her husband and a friend waited nearby in a motel room for word that it was over.

Most Americans are sympathetic with persons who must die a slow, lingering, painful death due to severe terminal illness. We can understand how, even when pain is controlled, the suffering that accompanies dying must also be addressed. For this reason a good argument can be made that doctors should assist in dying, in bringing about a good death, in the face of burgeoning medical technology (Cerne, 1990). For the most part this can be accomplished by passive euthanasia—by withholding or even withdrawing medical technology at the patient's request (Stanley, 1989). Both withholding and withdrawing are forms of taking responsibility for our technology. Keeping technology out of the dying process at the request of the patient and family is a way of honoring the primacy of human life and human values.

Mrs. Adkins' case, however, seems to have been unusual. She was only in the initial stages of Alzheimer's disease, and treatment technology was neither present nor imminent. There were to be many days and years ahead of her which she could still enjoy. Patients suffering far more than she struggle with the existential question of existence every day and still make up their minds to live (Mosley, 1990).

Mrs. Adkins' death at the hands of the "suicide machine" and Dr. Kevorkian raises many difficult questions. Should assisted suicide by doctors be legalized? Even if it were legal, is it moral? Does it differ from euthanasia? Should doctors be involved, considering their traditional commitments to healing by protecting and serving human life? These questions should be at the heart of public discussions about our duties to the sick and dying in a technological age. Most important, however, is the issue of whether Mrs. Adkins' suffering was sufficient to warrant legal and moral acceptance of her act. Does it not matter that patients must "suffer" (however that is to be defined) in order to request assisted suicide? Is dementia to be considered a terminal illness that would justify rational suicide or euthanasia?

Public discussion of such issues should be massive and include consideration of what sort of society we ought to be. Have we become so disjointed as a society that people feel the need to dispatch themselves early in a chronic disease rather than trust others to care for them, rather than subject themselves to possible violations of their values in nursing homes and hospitals after they become senile? Evidence suggests that there is a growing trend in elder suicide (Conwell et al., 1990, pp. 640–644). Will people increasingly feel threatened by high-technology hospitals where they are stripped of their values at the same time they are stripped of their clothing and put into the beds? Do we have to carry all sorts of lengthy legal documents on our person about our wishes regarding medical technology should we become ill or get in an accident?

THE RIGHT TO DIE

Societal concerns about rising health care costs, and anxieties about the economic burdens of a rapidly increasing older population, may lead to increased pressures for the mercy killing of those who no longer are capable of a minimal quality of life (see Binstock and Post, 1991). Indeed, euthanasia is already one of the most volatile ethical issues confronting medical practice today. Reviews of gradual changes in attitude among physicians themselves, or among traditionally strong interventionist services such as emergency medicine, demonstrate a growing acceptance of passive and even active, direct euthanasia (Sprung, 1990). (Physician-assisted suicide is seen as distinct from euthanasia, because the patient performs the life-terminating act, as did Janet Adkins in activating Dr. Kevorkian's machine). And because euthanasia is based on a model of patients' "rights," it appears to have growing acceptance in the population at large.

Euthanasia, that is, direct voluntary mercy killing, should be kept morally separate from the many laudable advances that have occurred in underlining the rights of patients to determine the treatments they desire and do not desire during the dying process, and to choose treatments at any time during life, not just while dying. The efforts of patient advocacy groups in sponsoring and supporting legislation and court deliberations have been outstanding. Increased use of state laws facilitating advance-directive instruments, including the living will and the durable power of attorney, will clarify the nature and extent of these rights. What is important to note is that the underlying motivation for the development of such instruments is the prevention of suffering (Mehling, 1988).

It is active euthanasia that American medicine resists, not passive euthanasia—that is, treatment withdrawal or refusal. Against the backdrop of reports about active euthanasia in the United States, and concomitant reports from the Netherlands, the American medical profession's official position remains solidly that of its traditional repugnance for directly causing or intending death. The American Medical Association (AMA) published its guidelines on withholding and withdrawing life-sustaining treatment in 1986:

> The social commitment of the physician is to sustain life and relieve suffering. Where the performance of one duty conflicts with the other, the choice of the patient should prevail. (American Medical Association, 1986, pp. 12–13)

This view represents an endorsement of passive rather than active euthanasia.

What the AMA rejects is a "right to die" which goes beyond withholding or withdrawing treatment. Without question, a major effort is under way to develop this form of the right to die (Meisel, 1989). A vigorous assertion of the right to active euthanasia was expressed, for example, by Joseph Fletcher, an early, continuous, and strong proponent of a right to die. Fletcher says: "Death control . . . is a matter of human dignity. Without it persons become puppets. To perceive this is to grasp the error lurking in the notion that life, as such, is the highest good" (Fletcher, 1974, p. 4). Margaret P. Battin even argued that it may be more humane to prefer direct killing, senicide, than to deny life-prolonging treatment to the demented elderly (Battin, 1987).

The strongest form of the argument that there is a right to active euthanasia or assisted suicide stems from purist notions of individual autonomy. Individuals, it is reasoned, have a right to active, direct euthanasia, first because they should not have to suffer at the hands of modern medical technology if they do not wish to do so, and second because we should honor their individual self-determination, even if we think it is wrongheaded. I will contest these arguments.

For individuals to control the circumstances of their own dying, it is argued, they must be empowered to request active, direct euthanasia. If individuals have such a right, it creates duties for caregivers and others to assist in a good death. Human beings are ethically obligated to bring about the good for others (Thomasma and Graber, 1990). But as I argue later, this obligation does not ground a duty to provide direct euthanasia, but rather a duty to provide adequate pain control and a personal extension of an individual caregiver into the suffering of another.

Many physicians are concerned, understandably, about community perceptions that they are involved in voluntary active euthanasia. Thus, Leon Kass presents a thoughtful articulation of what is owed a dying patient by the physician. He argues that humanity is owed humanity, not just "humaneness" (i.e., being merciful by killing the patient). Kass maintains that the very reason we are compelled to put animals out of their misery is that they are not human and thus demand from us some measure of humaneness. By contrast, human beings demand from us our humanity itself. This thesis, in turn, rests on the relationship "between the healer and the ill" as constituted, essentially, "even if only tacitly, around the desire of both to promote the wholeness of the one who is ailing" (Kass, 1989a, p. 1).

Kass's argument is eloquently summarized in his challenge to those who wish to respect the personhood and autonomy of patients:

> People who care for autonomy and dignity should try to reverse this dehumanization of the last stages of life, instead of giving dehumanization its final triumph by welcoming the desperate good-bye-to-all that is contained in one final plea for poison. (Kass, 1989b, p. 45)

PASSIVE EUTHANASIA: A REASONABLE ALTERNATIVE

Some forms of euthanasia practiced in the United States today are more acceptable than others (Thomasma, 1988; Thomasma and Graber, 1990). But is active, direct euthanasia the best way to support suffering persons (see MacKinnon, 1988)? When the physician and other caregivers in society approach a dying patient, is the option for terminating that life an important part of the care to be offered? Patients have complications that require palliative care that sometimes shortens the process of dying, yet physicians still maintain the traditional duty to respect the life of patients. If the physician or other caregiver is committed to preserving the life of the patient, is there an alternative to active euthanasia which will not neglect the suffering of that patient?

Dramatic changes in health care have also changed the personal and social ritual of dying. There has been an enormous increase in the technology of care. Where once a cold compress might have been applied and one's hands held, now all sorts of interventions are possible, from intravenous fluids and nutrition, nasogastric feeding tubes, tubes implanted directly in a vein or stomach for feeding (bypassing cancerous obstructions), blood products and agents to prevent clotting or bleeding, and cardiopulmonary resuscitation to experimental treatments such as advanced chemotherapeutic agents, radiologic implants, artificial hearts, and transplants of other organs.

With the increase in technology comes a corresponding increase in the institutionalization of care. Whereas formerly patients died at home in the midst of the family, relatives, and friends, now they die in hospitals. Almost 80 percent of those who die each year die in institutions. Many of the personal freedoms enjoyed by dying persons are lost as a result. Hospitals are excellent places to go if one wants to be cured of a disease, but they can be terrible places in which to die.

Increases in technology and institutionalization also engender a corresponding increase in the specialization of care. No one person attends to the dying patient. Often different services are stacked up like planes at a busy airport, waiting to attend the dying person. At risk, then, is the former freedom to control one's own dying process.

In our hospitals it is actually difficult to die. There is little possibility to maintain the personal and social ritual of dying. In a technology-intensive hospital, it is even difficult to sense that one is dying. The patient and the family have no clues about what will be the final event. The dying process is sometimes disrupted in favor of doing all one can to preserve life. Hence it is hard to assemble family and friends for a last conversation. How many persons have gone to and fro from the deathbeds of their relatives, wondering if each trip would be the last? Even if one knew that death was approaching, there was a diminished chance that last words could be spoken. This is true because the prolongation of the dying process, if it is successful and provides a few more good days, weeks, or months, usually terminates in a process of pain during which the patient is severely drugged.

Moreover, people's bodies die in pieces. First their kidneys might go, then their liver, then their heart, and finally their lungs. During this process, they have invited into their bodies all sorts of interventions, such as fluids, nutrition, antibiotics, surgeries of various sorts, respirators, and nasogastric feeding tubes. There is no one to preside over the moment of death, since the dying is spread out over so many moments.

Even though persons have always died in pieces—that is, their bodies have deteriorated or parts of the body have shut down—because of the social ritual and community support in the past, the person did not disintegrate from a metaphysical point of view. Each person was assured of support, convinced that loved ones were near and that a smooth transition to an afterlife would be provided by religious ritual attendant on their deathbeds.

Personal control of the dying process can be regained by appealing to a number of medical ethics principles rather than just to honoring the autonomy of the patient. Some of these have now been recognized in the law as well. One obvious principle is that of "informed consent." This standard originally applied to medical research, but in *Canterbury v. Spence* in 1972 it was applied by the District of Columbia Circuit Court to regular medical treatment (*Canterbury v. Spence*, 1972). The principle is that individuals have a right to decide about their own medical treatment and must have sufficient information and freedom to make that choice. As Russell McIntyre noted about a New Jersey Supreme Court adoption of the "objective prudent patient standard" in regard to informed consent, the obligation of providing information and being sure the patient is free to make the decision falls on the physician, and the requirement to pursue this obligation is linked to New Jersey's other supreme court judgments regarding the right to die (McIntyre, 1988). These judgments involve protection of the rights of patients to avoid abuse.

First, all patients have a right to refuse treatment, even if this refusal might lead to their death. Court cases, such as *In re Conroy* (1985) and *In re Jobes* (1987), have confirmed this right, even for incompetent patients. An incompetent patient does not lose the right to refuse treatment; the guardian or family member must speak for their wishes. Thus the family does not have a right to say what it would want so much as what the patient would prefer. This right of the patient perdures whether or not there is living-will legislation in his or her state. Of course, a living will strengthens the advance directive a patient gives about his or her care.

However, in what was characterized as a setback from the right to die movement, the Supreme Court of the State of Missouri forbade the withdrawal of artificial nutrition and hydration through a gastrostomy in the case of Nancy Cruzan, who lay in a permanent vegetative state for five years as a result of an automobile accident (*Cruzan v. Harmon*, 1989). She was then 30 years old. If the feeding had continued, she might have been expected to live another thirty years in that condition. Her family had argued that she did not wish to live in such a condition. Their argument was based on a "somewhat serious conversation" in which Nancy had indicated that if sick or injured she would not want to have her life continued unless she could live "halfway normally." A trial court found this sufficient evidence that she would not want to live maintained only on artificial food and hydration, and ordered the state employees caring for her in the Mount Vernon State Hospital to carry out the request of her legal guardians to withdraw the fluids and nutrition.

But on appeal, the Missouri Supreme Court brushed aside the nearly one hundred court cases in twenty states, and the living-will statutes in thirty-eight states, including Missouri itself. The majority opinion (4–3) held that the constitutional right to privacy is not expansive enough to apply to lifesaving treatment. The overwhelming majority of the previous court cases that the Missouri court considered had been decided in favor of the right to die. These cases had also affirmed the role of families or other decision-makers, who are able to say, in the absence of written preferences from patients, that the patient would not have wanted the treatments in question. But the Missouri court considered that euphemisms made their way to the fore in these other cases, particularly the construct that by withdrawing fluids and nutrition, the patient died of the underlying disease.

The U.S. Supreme Court's decision in this case (*Cruzan v. Director, Missouri Department of Health*, 1990) makes it clear that competent patients have a liberty to refuse treatment, and that medically delivered fluids and nutrition are to be considered refusable interventions. The decision indirectly affirmed the need for living wills and advance directives. Yet it also affirmed the right of states to require "clear and convincing evidence" of an incompetent patient's wishes. In this way it counterbalanced a pure autonomy approach with an interest in protecting the vulnerable from harm. Hospitals are now making efforts to help patients execute living wills and/or a durable power of attorney, not only to protect the autonomy of individuals, but also out of self-interest regarding the cost of keeping incompetent patients alive in the absence of previously expressed wishes.

One problem in the Missouri case was with the specificity of wishes. In this regard, the court built upon an earlier and less restrictive judgment handed down in New York regarding Mary O'Connor. The decision in New York is considered less restrictive because it did not deny the right of patients to express advance directives or that the family might have a legitimate role in witnessing those directives, but that O'Connor had made any specific reference to fluids and nutrition in her wishes. She was 77, a widow, with two daughters who were practical nurses. During her later years, she frequently had to confront issues of life prolongation with relatives and her husband. The daughters and friends were able to testify to her constant and explicit desire never to "be a burden to anyone," "not to lose my dignity"; that it was "monstrous" to keep someone alive using machinery when they are "not going to get any better." She held that people who were suffering very badly should be allowed to die. Several times she told Helen, one of her daughters, that if she became ill and could not take care of herself, she would not want her life to be sustained artificially (*Medical Ethics Advisor*, 1989). A trial court approved removal of fluids and nutrition after her progressive deterioration from a series of strokes. She was in a geriatric institute at the time. The appellate court affirmed that ruling, but when the institute went to the New York Court of Appeals, it issued a surprise ruling. After affirming the ideal situation of having advance directives from the patient herself, or a living will (which is not yet legal in New York), and acknowledging that repeated oral expressions are important, the rulings of the lower courts were overturned because the patient's statements, as expressed by family and friends, were not clear about application for withdrawing fluids and nutrition (p. 15).

The Society for the Right to Die commented on this New York case with respect to the role of the family:

> The underlying assumption is that to permit ending treatment without clear and convincing evidence would lead to abuse of the vulnerable elderly. Other courts and authorities . . . have strongly held that decision-making when the patient is incompetent is best discharged by family members who know and care for the patient, rather than health care provider or courts, to whom she may be a stranger. (*Medical Ethics Advisor*, 1989, pp. 15–16)

The court's position is that there is nothing more than conjecture about whether O'Connor would have wanted the fluids and nutrition withdrawn. One suspects, however, that a more conservative concern about many vulnerable individuals has now surfaced. This concern has a deep background, including the Nazi experience. Yet the question remains, how specific can or must individuals be about the future contingent possibilities of their health? It seems sufficient to take the "family principle" seriously, that lacking any other data, families are the best interpreters of their loved one's wishes, unless, of course, the family itself is judged incompetent to speak for their loved one for one reason or another.

Second, in addition to the living will and other forms of controlling the dying process, a way to control one's dying is found in Do Not Resuscitate (DNR) orders. Patients have a right to require DNR orders in the hospital. These orders mean that no resuscitation efforts will be made during the dying process should one's heart and breathing stop. In fact, cardiopulmonary resuscitation was never intended for dying patients. Rather, it was meant for emergency interventions when someone suddenly had a heart attack or respiratory arrest. Given the right to refuse treatment, patients and their families may also refuse other interventions such as antibiotics, nasogastric feeding tubes, intravenous fluids and nutrition, and the like (Shannon and Walter, 1988; Lynn, 1987). In the case of dying patients, all treatments should be seen as optional, especially if they might prolong the dying process.

Third, for those patients who have left few or no instructions about what they would like to have done during their dying process, physicians and families may employ the distinction between ordinary and extraordinary means. Ordinary means, in Pope Pius xii's early formulation of this distinction, were those that represented little or no burden on the patient. Extraordinary means were those that presented a burden on the patient or family. Economic considerations were possible in this schema. The distinction fell on hard times later, when persons began to make of it a normative category: Ordinary means was to signify those usual medical treatments that were required, extraordinary means to signify those unusual treatments that would be optional. Because of this confusion between normative meanings for the ordinary/extraordinary distinction and the original meaning of burdensomeness, today most ethicists and the courts prefer to use the principle of proportionality. According to this principle, only those interventions should be used which can demonstrate a proportionately higher benefit to the patient than burden. If one is thirsty but cannot drink water, then intravenous fluids make sense, since the benefit outweighs the burden. If one is dying, and fluids and nutrition merely prolong that dying process, then the interventions are judged disproportionate to the outcome and are optional. In this instance, food and water are delivered through a medical technology, and they are called fluids and nutrition to make the distinction between the normal way of receiving nourishment through the mouth and a medical intervention.

Fourth, the principle of double effect can be used to control pain even if by this control one's respirations would be depressed and one would die. According to the principle of double effect, one action (using very high doses of morphine to control pain) can produce two effects (control of pain and suffering and depressed respirations or death). Even though the second effect is foreseen, it is not intended. Thus, it is not necessary to keep a dying person in a state of suffering and anguish from pain out of fear that the high doses of pain control medication might kill him or her. The first duty of a physician is to control pain, and the second is not to impose his or her values about suffering on the patient (Pellegrino, 1982). The obligation to control pain and address suffering is a major force at this point. Health care professionals themselves suffer by opening themselves to the suffering of dying patients. They expose themselves to their own vulnerability, their own losses, and their own wounds. It is not just a matter of feelings of inadequacy in the presence of their own helplessness. It is a matter of sharing in the fundamental finitude of human nature (Latimer, 1990).

Finally, referral to hospice care makes eminent sense when one is dying (if the disease permits). In hospice care, cruelty is avoided, as are all forms of medical technology which might unduly prolong dying (Lamers, 1986). Even though the case is hopeless, the community can provide the support and personal attention a dying person commands as a duty from the rest of us.

Keeping a person alive at all costs is a form of biological idolatry. This idolatry denies the finitude of human existence in favor of a Faustian adventure at the expense of the dying person. If that person wishes to participate in this adventure, he or she may sign on of course. But at present, the default mode should not be the assumption that care can only be delivered by high-technology medicine. Personal healing is a ministry of persons, not of technology. Further, persons should not be subject to the loss of control over their dying to technology, or to other persons, however high-minded those other considerations or persons might be. The dying person in our society deserves at least this much.

Although all beings should be valued by us, and their integrity preserved as far as possible, when a tragic choice is forced on us, it is far easier to decide about applying a medical technology or withholding it altogether based on values constructed by a patient over a lifetime than on a "value-less" field presented by the embryo or newborn. That is why the abortion debate has divided us so politically, and much more so, than debates about the living will and other forms of controlling the dying process (though the latter, too, have been vigorously argued). Honoring the values of the individual as part of decisions to be made about them, once they are incompetent, is the primary way we can respect their inherent dignity. If they are dying, we should never strip them of the lifetime of choices their values represent. In this way the

U.S. Supreme Court decision in *Cruzan* violates some of our most deeply held feelings about the ability of a family to express the value history of the patient. As there are a large number of demented elderly who have never made their explicit wishes known about their care, employing the family's potential to help make decisions about their care on the basis of their values is essential.

Attorney James Bopp has argued that the *Cruzan* decision by the Missouri Supreme Court denotes a trend away from creating more privacy rights and from delegating authority to third parties. Clearly at risk in the decision by the U.S. Supreme Court is the right of surrogates to speak for incapacitated individuals. But this risk betrays an even deeper one, the right "to control medical decisions affecting our own bodies," in the words of Fenella Rouse, J.D., director of the Society for the Right to Die (Weinstein, 1989, p. 9).

While Rouse argues the by-now accepted view of most medical ethicists that surrogates are empowered to make decisions for individuals when they become incompetent, as Nancy Cruzan's parents did on her behalf, the general counsel of the National Right-to-Life Committee thinks that the burden must fall on the parents to prove a "specific and concrete" right to assert a right of privacy for their daughter. As he noted, "We can't establish a rule where life can be ended by third parties" (Weinstein, 1989, p. 9). Bopp (1990) has carefully argued for a legal obligation to provide care in the absence of strict advance directives. His concern is that once persons become incompetent, our society might dispatch them on the basis of questionable quality-of-life judgments. In his view, the law should continue to protect such vulnerable individuals from the judgments of others, even if these others are close family members, like Cruzan's parents. Will it be easier to use a simple method of dispatching those persons whose care costs too much, or who are now considered to be a burden on society, like the aged and the poor, than to address their suffering, which sometimes is overwhelming even for the most dedicated caregivers?

While I stress the right of surrogates to act on previously expressed wishes of the patient, this assertion may not adequately confront the problems often faced by geriatric specialists when doctors must act in the best interests of many elderly patients who have left no valid documents expressing their preferences and who have no identifiable surrogates to speak for their values. For this reason I favor a public policy stand that requires advance directives at various times during one's life, and especially upon entering any health care or nursing care institution.

A position of solid commitment to the value of human life, even that which may not be a human person as we normally understand personhood, produces the safest insurance against bigotry, repression, neo-Nazism, and murder. There is much to be said of this position.

CONTROLLING LIFE-PROLONGING TECHNOLOGIES: THE NEW THREAT OF "CLEAR AND GROWING EVIDENCE"

Controlling life-prolonging technologies is an important aspect of the larger problem of directing technology to human aims. Nowhere is that more apparent than in the application of medical technology and its various interventions to the dying patient (among whom I number those in advanced stages of dementia). Not surprisingly, studies have confirmed that it is not the technology but the care persons receive which determines their well-being and, in the case of the dying patient, the protection of their human spirit to the end.

Every person should have the right not to be subject to the products of human imagination without his or her consent. No person should be subject to technologies without some increased benefit to quality of life. This is what we mean by saying that the value of human life must be respected. In the Judeo-Christian heritage of Western civilization, we believe that God made persons a little less than the angels. Crowned with dignity and honor, human beings are greater than their inventions.

Is it good public policy to continue to insist that individuals make specific and concrete advance directives? After all, how much future forecasting are most human beings able to do? Not being sophisticated about health care is a major danger in our society today, since we are able to lose our rights over what will be done to us when we become incompetent. Yet most people are occupied with the tasks of daily life, so much so that they neglect to fill out a living will or other advance directive, even in states where these documents are legal and encouraged.

Because of such difficulties, present discussion about advance directives veers in the wrong direction. The court decisions all focus on the specificity of advance wishes instead of on the default mode of modern medicine. The default mode of modern medicine is that—absent any directives to the contrary—all individuals want "everything possible done to save their lives." Evidence exists through surveys that this is just not so. Most people, on reaching certain states of neurological impairment, do not want their lives prolonged in those conditions, even if they are not, strictly speaking, considered to be states of "dying." This is, in fact, the basis of the argument of Nancy Cruzan's parents to respect her values and allow her to die.

The default mode of modern medicine ought to be the reverse. Rather than a treatment mode, *it should be that absent any advance directives to the contrary*, in specified states of neurological impairment, *individuals will not receive medical interventions* (including medically delivered fluids and nutrition) *to prolong their lives.*

A public policy embodying this default mode would ensure that individuals make out living wills, advance directives, or durable powers of attorney, if they feel strongly about having their lives prolonged. It would save society the monies now being spent on what many of us would call "useless therapy" in what for lack of a better term can only be called "feeding wards." Furthermore, it would protect the dignity of individuals who, for one reason or another, fall into states of neuro-logical impairment or other chronic and debilitating states and who have not informed us specifically enough about what to do with their care.

But what should we do with Bopp's contention that when patients have not directly and specifically let us know their wishes, the law should protect the "inestimable value of life"? Bopp interprets this protection as "ensuring that the patient receives beneficial medical care" (Bopp, 1990, p. 601). He further charges that the position state-ment of the Society for the Right to Die overcomes "the legal obligation to provide care" by permitting a surrogate who knows the patient to refuse such care based on "quality of life considerations." He finds such overruling of the legal obligation morally repugnant.

In addition to the suggestion just made that a change should be made in the default mode of medicine when certain conditions destroy the ability of patients to interact spiritually and materially in human life, I also suggest that Bopp's identification of beneficial medical care with continued intervention is faulty. The judgment of what is best for patients should be protected in the law. But this protection should be one that supports decision-making on a case-by-case basis with the family and physicians who know the patient. The state's interests in protecting life, as Oberman argues, should be confined to protecting the autonomy of persons and their loved ones in making appropriate decisions, and judging whether such decisions are made by competent persons. It should not be interpreted as a mandate to intervene when-ever an individual's act puts his or her life in potential danger (Ober-man, 1989).

PROTECTING THE MOST VULNERABLE: TWO PRINCIPLES OF CLINICAL ETHICS

In the end, the only way to protect the most vulnerable patients is to act on the basis of their values, or their values as expressed by the surrogates who know them the best. Otherwise, patients with severe dementia, and all of us, will be at risk of being stripped of our most precious possession, the values we stood for all during our lives.

Yet, in the wake of the *Cruzan* decision by the United States Supreme Court, physicians will be tempted to rely on additional legal data when making medical decisions about incompetent patients. This is unfortunate. Sometimes it is tragic. As already noted, the Court chose not to rely on verbally expressed wishes of patients prior to the event that made them incompetent; nor, and this is most unfortunate, did it choose to rely on the judgment of surrogates, like Nancy Cruzan's parents, to convey and interpret her wishes. It determined that states have a right to require more "clear and convincing" evidence of the patient's wishes than Nancy's parents were able to provide.

As I have argued, it is a good social policy for society to protect its most vulnerable citizens. But the protection must cut both ways. On the one hand, it is important not to slip into a Nazi-like society in which the least competent persons—the demented and debilitated, the retarded, the defective newborns—are summarily taken away and euthanized out of a twisted sense of "compassion." This is the most extreme form of involuntary euthanasia. There is no real danger in the near future of American medicine conducting its affairs under the control of the state in this fashion.

Yet the "slipperly slope" argument acquires its force from the initial steps taken toward such a downward slide of ethics and social policy. And the first steps, so the argument goes, are taken when society permits the destruction of innocent human life. First the fetus, then the aged and incompetent patient, and then patients in persistent vegetative states and permanent comas are "helped to die." Such "help" is considered a euphemism for early dispatching of those who either never could or can no longer speak for themselves. These beings must receive protection, more so than others who are competent and can still express their determination about medical treatments.

A clinical ethical principle is born of concern for the severely demented and other highly vulnerable persons (Thomasma, in press). The greater the degree of the patient's incompetence, and the less the invasiveness of medical procedure, the more formal the quality of the individual's preferences which should be required. Patients with persistent vegetative states or permanent comas or end-stage Alzheimer's disease, for example, are now unable to speak for themselves. They have a high degree of incompetence. If the therapeutic plan turns on the question of withholding and withdrawing fluids and nutrition, these are considered less invasive procedures than using respirators and cardiopulmonary resuscitation. Withholding and withdrawing nutrition and hydration from such patients on the basis of their previous statements, according to this first ethical principle, can be done, but it requires a very explicit, "clear and convincing" form of evidence. One form might be a living will or written advance directive. Informal discussion with relatives may be insufficient. Legal documentation is to be preferred.

On the other hand, dementia sufferers must be protected from another sort of harm. This is the harm brought to us courtesy of modern, high-technology health care. For the most part we are able to control this technology by directing it to good human ends. Healing and curing patients are good examples. When highly technical means for curing individuals are employed, however, there is a danger that the means will begin to obscure the ends. This is especially true when the intervention has "frozen" persons in states that normally would have led to their deaths, just as modern medicine can freeze embryos on their way to their lives.

When individuals are severely demented, we must take responsibility for the technology employed in keeping them alive, far from the normal interactive, personal life they once enjoyed. They cannot be cured. They cannot be healed. Such patients are controlled by the whims of others who perceive themselves as protectors of human life.

Arising from this additional concern to protect the vulnerable, then, is a second ethical principle. How may we protect incompetent patients from being at the mercy of others? How may we control the enthusiasms of the life-prolongers-at-all-costs? How should we properly direct our medical technology? This contrasting clinical ethics principle might be expressed as follows: The greater the permanent assault on the quality of personal, interactive human life, the less formal the quality of consent is required in order to withhold and withdraw medical treatment that might prolong life in such uncertain conditions, and the greater might be the reliance on the patient's preferences as expressed informally to the family or as constructed by the family from the patient's value history.

Physicians and patients must now develop the importance of the second clinical ethics principle, so that the flexibility and dialogue about values which are so essential to the doctor-patient relationship are not lost in a legal quagmire of documentation. There is still time to propose legislation in states that have no guidelines about decisions for incompetent patients which would name the family and other significant parties as default decision-makers with the managing physicians. This legislation should be proposed as an essential means for protecting the most vulnerable patients from the harm of overemployment of our life-prolonging technology.

I have argued that mercy killing of the demented elderly should not be an option in our society. There are better ways to honor the dignity of personal human lives whose personhood has almost entirely vanished. Passive euthanasia is one of these ways. I have tried to spell out how a program of passive euthanasia could honor the wishes of individuals who later spiral into a kind of personal oblivion. When wishes are not present, I have also argued for the right of families to construct a patient's value history that would help determine what he or she might want done.

Even though each individual has a right to decide how his or her own life is to be valued, it is wise that society itself controls the urge to kill oneself or others. While a good death is a benefit to all of us, the duty to help bring it about can be fulfilled through loving care of individuals, proper control of our medical technology, and community support through hospice programs. Rarely, if ever, should we resort to actively killing others, even at their own request. Because of their special vulnerability, this is especially true of the demented elderly.

REFERENCES

American Medical Association, Council on Ethical and Judicial Affairs. (1986). Withholding and withdrawing life-prolonging medical treatment. In *Current Opinions of the Council on Ethical and Judicial Affairs of the American Medical Association*, pp. 12–13. Chicago: American Medical Association.

Battin, M.P. (1987). Age rationing and the just distribution of health care: is there a duty to die? In T.M. Smeeding, ed., *Should Medical Care Be Rationed by Age?* pp. 69–94. Totowa, N.J.: Rowman and Littlefield.

Binstock, R.H., and Post, S.G., eds. (1991). *Too Old for Health Care? Controversies in Medicine, Law, Economics, and Ethics*. Baltimore, Md.: Johns Hopkins University Press.

Bopp, J. (1990). Reconciling autonomy and the value of life. *Journal of the American Geriatrics Society, 38*(6):600–602.

Canterbury v. Spence (1972). 464 F.2d. 772 (D.C. Cir.), *certiorari denied*, 409 U.S. 1064, 93 S.Ct. 560, 43 L.Ed.2d 518.

Cerne, F. (1990). Mercy or murder? physician's role in suicide spurs debate. *American Hospital Association News, 26*(26):1, 5.

Conwell, Y., Rotenberg, M., and Caine, E.D. (1990). Completed suicide at age 50 and over. *Journal of the American Geriatrics Society, 38*(6):640–644.

Cruzan v. Director, Missouri Department of Health (1990). U.S. Supreme Court, June 25, No. 88-1503.

Cruzan v. Harmon (1989). 760 S.W.2d 408 (Mo., 1988), *certiorari granted*, 109 S.Ct. 3240 (#88-1503).

Fletcher, J. (1974). Indicators of humanhood: the inquiry matures. *Hastings Center Report, 4*(6):4–7.

In re Conroy (1985). 98 N.J. 321, 486 A.2d 1209.

In re Jobes (1987). 108 N.J. 394, 529 A.2d 434.

Kass, L. (1989a). Arguments against active euthanasia by doctors found at medicine's core. *Kennedy Institute of Ethics Newsletter, 3*(January):1–3, 6.

Kass, L. (1989b). Neither for love nor money: why doctors must not kill. *Public Interest, 94:*25–46.

Lamers, W.M. (1986). Hospice care in North America. In S.B. Day, ed., *Cancer, Stress and Death* (2d ed.), pp. 133–148. New York: Plenum Press.

Latimer, E.J. (1990). The pain of cancer: helping patients and families: II. *Humane Medicine, 6*(3):189–192.

Lynn, J., ed. (1987). *By No Extraordinary Means.* Bloomington, Ind.: Indiana University Press.

MacKinnon, K. (1988). Active euthanasia: a "cop-out"? *Journal of Palliative Care, 4:*110.

McIntyre, R. (1988). Comment: perspective on medical ethics. *Info Trends: Medicine, Law and Ethics, 4*(1):5–6.

Medical Ethics Advisor (1989). O'Connor case highlights problem of incompetent patient with no living will. *5*(1):13–16.

Mehling, A. (1988). Living wills: preventing suffering or a deadly contract? *State Government News* (December):14–15.

Meisel, A. (1989). *The Right to Die.* Colorado Springs, Colo.: Wiley Law Publications.

Mosley, M. (1990). Is death ever better than life? *Ethics Rounds, 1*(6):2.

Oberman, M. (1989). Withdrawal of life support: individual autonomy against alleged state interests in preserving life. *Loyola University of Chicago Law Journal, 20*(3):797–818.

Pellegrino, E.D. (1982). The clinical ethics of pain management in the terminally ill. *Hospital Formulary, 17*(11):1493–1496.

Shannon, T., and Walter, J. (1988). The PVS patient and the forgoing/withdrawing of medical nutrition and hydration. *Theological Studies, 49:*623–647.

Sprung, C.L. (1990). Changing attitudes and practices in forgoing life-sustaining treatments. *Journal of the American Medical Association, 263*(16): 2211–2215.

Stanley, J.M., ed. (1989). The Appleton consensus: suggested international guidelines for decisions to forgo medical treatment. *Journal of Medical Ethics, 15:*129–136.

Thomasma, D.C. (1988). The range of euthanasia. *Bulletin of the American College of Surgeons, 73*(August):4–13.

Thomasma, D.C. (In press). Ethical aspects of geriatric care. In E. Calkins, A.B. Ford, and P.R. Katz, eds., *The Practice of Geriatrics* (2d ed.). Philadelphia: W.B. Saunders.

Thomasma, D.C., and Graber, G.C. (1990). *Euthanasia: Toward an Ethical Social Policy.* New York: Continuum.

Weinstein, M. (1989). U.S. Supreme Court to hear first case involving right-to-die. *ACP Observer, 2*(7):9.

9

EUTHANASIA
IN ALZHEIMER'S DISEASE?

Margaret P. Battin

Ought euthanasia be practiced for persons with advanced dementia? Although the issue of euthanasia is a topic of increasingly heated social debate, already tending to polarize those who support it as voluntary "aid-in-dying" and those who reject it as medical "killing," what is said about active euthanasia on *both* sides is severely challenged by the question of euthanasia in Alzheimer's disease. Whether euthanasia may or should be practiced in Alzheimer's is not an easy moral or social-policy question to answer, as I shall try to show, even if one finds the answers to moral and policy questions about euthanasia comparatively simple in other contexts.

   In showing why the question of euthanasia in Alzheimer's is so difficult to answer, I'd like to survey the three most prevalent arguments for euthanasia in general, the arguments from autonomy, from mercy, and from justice (Battin, 1987), and show what is problematic about each. All three yield indeterminate answers. Although none of these conventional arguments for euthanasia seems to be effective in the specific circumstances of Alzheimer's, the considerations they raise also fail to produce effective arguments against euthanasia. But a philosophically indeterminate position of this sort seems a luxury, given the literally millions of people potentially directly affected by social policies that might be formulated on the basis of such discussions. Given these inconclusive results, I then turn to look at what is usually the principal argument against euthanasia—the "slippery-slope" argument —and find that it gives equally disturbing results. Finally, I look briefly at the question this situation poses: How can one formulate social

policy in such a sensitive matter as this, when background philosophical considerations do not seem to prove much help?

What I shall be considering here is whether *active* euthanasia may
be practiced on persons with advanced Alzheimer's—that is, direct
killing, performed in the paradigmatic case by a physician as a medical
procedure intended to produce death. It is without question the case
that in terminal illness we already often practice what philosophers
(but not doctors or the general public) call passive euthanasia: the withholding or withdrawal of treatment that would otherwise prolong life,
thus "allowing" the patient to die. We also often practice a form of
life curtailment involving the overadministration of morphine; in these
cases, it is usually argued, the intention is to relieve pain, and the
respiratory suppression that results in death is a foreseen but unin-
tended consequence. While both of these may and do occur in Alzheimer's, I shall be considering neither here: I am concerned with whether
directly produced death, produced because of the Alzheimer's rather
than for other reasons, is morally warranted. To be sure, any discussion of the moral issues in euthanasia rejects the categorical argument
that killing or causing the death of human beings is always wrong;
pointing to practices often regarded as morally acceptable, including
killing in self-defense, just war, abortion, and capital punishment, such
a discussion presupposes that if any of these practices are morally
permissible, it must be argued, not assumed, that killing in euthanasia
cannot also be so.

THE PHILOSOPHICAL ARGUMENTS CONCERNING EUTHANASIA, AS APPLIED TO ADVANCED DEMENTIA

THE ARGUMENT FROM AUTONOMY

In contemporary defenses of active euthanasia, it is often argued
that the right to determine the character and timing of one's own death,
wherever doing so is possible, is a basic human right, grounded in
fundamental rights of self-determination and autonomy generally. Such
autonomy rights include all choices that are self-respecting only and
do not seriously damage the interests or violate the rights of others,
and certainly include, it is argued, rights of choice in matters so profound and intimately personal as deciding whether to continue to live
or to die. On this view, a course of action one knowingly and voluntarily chooses, provided it does not harm others, is one to which a
person has at least one and perhaps two sorts of rights: the negative
right not to be interfered with in the performance of the action and
perhaps in addition the positive right to be aided in or provided with
means for accomplishing the action. Of course, there may be grounds

for interference with exercise of this right either when it is chosen in an irrational, impaired way or when the interests of other parties would be jeopardized (say, those of minor children who would be left unsupported), but these circumstances are typically irrelevant in choices concerning euthanasia in Alzheimer's. On the argument from autonomy, the patient who knowingly and voluntarily elects death in preference to a medical situation such as Alzheimer's ought not be interrupted in any attempt to commit suicide and may even have claim to positive aid in physician-assisted suicide or physician-performed euthanasia. By and large, suicide by the Alzheimer's patient is possible only just after diagnosis or in the comparatively early stages of the disease, when he or she is still able to form and act on a plan and is likely to have access to means of suicide; active euthanasia could of course be performed at any point, though the issue I wish to address here is euthanasia in the late stages of the disease.

But is it meaningful at all to speak of autonomous choice in Alzheimer's? Can euthanasia be voluntary, the product of informed, free choice, in Alzheimer's? Given that Alzheimer's eventually involves complete deterioration of all cognitive skills, including the capacity to conceptualize, predict, understand information, deliberate about a matter, reason, or perform any sort of planning, it would seem that an Alzheimer's patient, at least in the advanced stages of dementia, could hardly *choose* euthanasia. After all, for such a choice to be fully enough informed to count as voluntary, the person must be able to understand not only the medical procedures actually used to produce death, but also the abstract notion of the transition from life to death. But while an advanced Alzheimer's patient may exhibit some behavior that looks like choosing in certain simple contexts—using a red crayon rather than a green one when coloring, for example, or sitting down or getting up from a chair—we do not suppose that these actions involve choice in any robust way or that they are anything more than simple responses to stimuli. We certainly do not think that such actions provide real evidence of abstract choice.

On the other hand, it would seem that choices of euthanasia governing the advanced Alzheimer's patient must be recognized as voluntary if they are made by the person while still competent and recorded in an advance-directive document such as a living will. The living will provides legally valid evidence (in most U.S. states) of a person's choices about treatment after she becomes incompetent. (Feminine pronoun has been used because, statistically, most patients are female.) To be sure, living-will declarations at the current moment in the United States cannot contain provisions concerning active euthanasia; in the Netherlands, in contrast, where euthanasia is legally tolerated, at least one standard living-will form does contain a provision permitting the request of active euthanasia, and we can imagine legislation permitting such choices in this country too. Of course, the living will brings with it various problems, among them that the signer of it may not correctly foresee the range of medical problems to occur in her future, that one may fluctuate in and out of competence and hence in and out of being subject to the provisions of one's own living will, or that one can revoke one's own living will after becoming no longer competent but cannot then later reexecute it. Nevertheless, the living will, which functions by recognizing precedent autonomy, is designed to expand the range of choices a person can make about herself: It gives legal force to choices that will take effect after that person is no longer currently capable of making any choice at all. If that person knew she might develop Alzheimer's and chose—with full information, and perfectly voluntarily—to request euthanasia should that occur, it is argued, this choice ought to be respected.

But does the living will actually represent a voluntary choice of the Alzheimer's patient? After all, the person whom this choice now concerns—the one perhaps to be put to death as a result of this choice, if euthanasia has been requested—can no longer understand the choice or reenact making it; indeed, the severely demented person cannot even remember making this profoundly important choice. After all, the choice was made by a long-distant version of herself, whom she no longer even remembers being. Can we actually say that she made this choice? Since in the United States only choices resulting in earlier death by withholding or withdrawing treatment are currently recognized, not choices employing active euthanasia, and since physicians, family members, payers, and others rarely object to choices to withhold or withdraw in severe dementia, the philosophical issue of the legitimacy of the advance directive is rarely raised. Nevertheless, the same issue seems to become much more pressing in the case of a highly contentious provision like a request for active euthanasia. Is it plausible to say that this person, the one who is now severely demented and has no awareness of her previous advance directive, knowingly and voluntarily requests to be killed? If it is not plausible, is there convincing reason for recognizing such a choice?

But then, can we actually say that she did not make this choice? It was her hand that put the pen to the paper, signing it; it was she who discussed it with her lawyer and relatives; it was she who was the legal agent employing a recognized legal instrument for effecting her own choice concerning the very circumstance in which she now finds herself. Choice is *always* choice about one's own future, though the time gap between present and future may be longer or shorter and the conditions more or less different. Only by adopting a Humean or Parfitean account of the self, in which there is no genuine continuity of person over time but only a set of overlapping bundles or person-stages, can we so radically divorce the present patient from her own former self as to say it is not *her* choice. She has changed, and changed dramatically, to be sure, but it is still she, we are inclined to say, who wrote the directive. After all, if it wasn't she who executed the directive, what other person did it?

The difference between these two conceptions is what Ronald Dworkin describes as the difference in conceiving of the Alzheimer's patient as "a demented person" or as "a person who has become demented" (Dworkin, 1986, p. 4). If we employ the former view, we give primary weight to current choices, allowing them to supersede prior ones (as, for example, in revoking a living will); on the latter, we give primary weight to the choices of the previously undemented person. Dworkin favors recognizing precedent rather than current autonomy in severe dementia, primarily because the value of autonomy lies in the way "autonomy makes each of us responsible for shaping his own life according to some coherent and distinctive sense of character, conviction, and interests" (p. 8); what is essential is the integrity of a person's life plan. This may be a reasonable policy proposal, but it does not really answer the philosophical question: Ought we recognize precedent autonomy in these extreme cases where the agent can no longer recognize her former self, or is autonomy here, if possible at all, always necessarily contemporary?

Can euthanasia in advanced Alzheimer's be voluntary? This, as we said, is not an easy question to answer, and even the sophisticated legal device of the living will, intended to cover circumstances of later incompetence precisely such as these, does not decide the philosophical question.

THE ARGUMENT FROM MERCY

Even though it is not clear whether euthanasia in advanced Alzheimer's can be voluntary, can it nevertheless be a gesture of mercy? Traditional arguments for euthanasia have often been arguments from mercy: that euthanasia is morally permissible when it is the only effective way to relieve a patient's pain or suffering and to spare the patient an otherwise agonizing death. Thus, regardless of whether euthanasia in advanced Alzheimer's can be voluntary, it is still open to question whether it might be legitimized, or perhaps even morally mandated, on grounds of mercy. This is not a question of the sufferings of others, especially family members who serve as principal caregivers, but of the sufferings of the Alzheimer's victim herself.

After all, while the early Alzheimer's patient can often still function fairly well, it is a long road downhill, and the advanced Alzheimer's patient's sufferings seem to be extreme. She loses her capacities for effective function in the world; she is increasingly bewildered by her circumstances; and she loses her capacity for interaction with family and friends, even those closest to her. She cannot read, think, play any game, or converse with anyone; and she cannot, as the traditional stereotype of benign old age would have it, sit in a rocking chair sifting through her memories of youth. Hers is a world without meaning, without purpose or project, without affectional ties. This is the condition the Dutch call *entluistering*, the "effacement" or complete eclipse of human personality, and for the Dutch, *entluistering* rather than pain is a primary reason for choices of euthanasia. Worse still, in those forms of Alzheimer's which involve paranoid delusions, the patient's experience may be peopled with creatures and situations or horrendously threatening sorts, but whose patterns she cannot predict and whose terms she cannot understand well enough to escape or accept. In some cases, dementia may be a kind of ongoing nightmare, full of shadows and threats that do not vanish when one wakes. Thus it looks as though euthanasia in advanced Alzheimer's might be warranted on grounds of mercy, whether or not it is voluntarily requested, because the mental suffering it involves may be so great.

But does the argument from mercy really succeed in Alzheimer's? We are often reluctant to speak of suffering where there is no self-aware subject of experiences; if this is so, the Alzheimer's victim cannot be said to be suffering. True, as an organism with a nervous system, the Alzheimer's victim, like other persons and also like animals, can of course feel pain, but pain is not to be confused with the distinctive kind of suffering the loss of cognitive function is said to produce. But does it? Does a person whose life is void of meaningful activity or important interpersonal contact thereby suffer? Or it is rather that her sensorium merely includes isolated, unconnected, uninterpreted sensory experiences but no cognitive awareness or experience of what she is missing? But if she has no awareness of what she is missing, she cannot suffer, anymore than one's pet dog experiences suffering from being unable to talk or do arithmetic or from being unable to plan for its own future. Even the demented patient with paranoid delusions, if she no longer has any sense of self, cannot suffer, it would seem, since there is no self there to whom these awful experiences happen; they occur, but in a mental void. But if these things are true and we take the having of a sense of self—that self-awareness often counted as distinctively human and as presupposed by the very notion of person—as prerequisite for suffering, then as the deterioration of Alzheimer's advances, the potential for suffering decreases. Paradoxically, it might seem, the greater the patient's losses, the weaker her claim to euthanasia on grounds of mercy.

The traditional argument for euthanasia on grounds of mercy points to physical pain and emotional suffering, but the former is irrelevant in the case of Alzheimer's and it is not clear whether the latter can occur. It is of course true that an Alzheimer's patient might have some untreatable coexisting medical condition about which the question of euthanasia because of intractable pain might be raised, but then this is not a question of euthanasia because of Alzheimer's and would have only tangential bearing on the million persons with severe Alzheimer's; the two to three million more with milder, though progressive, Alzheimer's; and indeed the rest of us, who, if we live to age 85, stand a one in four chance of developing it. But this just raises the question all over again: Do we not fear developing Alzheimer's because we do not want to suffer in this way?

If neither considerations of choice nor considerations of mercy will decide whether euthanasia should be performed for Alzheimer's patients, how then should we develop social policy in this very difficult matter? What about the argument that to keep such people alive defies any defensible principle of distributive justice—in other words, that to keep such people alive is a waste?

THE ISSUE OF JUSTICE

It is also often popularly argued that the expenditure of funds to care for Alzheimer's victims is a "waste." This is a form of distributive argument; it is based on the assumption that there are other more defensible distributions of health care and that it would be more just to allocate these resources to other parties with stronger claims to them than to have them consumed by Alzheimer's patients who are already severely demented and will never recover. While the cruder forms of the popular argument rarely spell out what distributive arrangement ought to be considered more just, what sorts of claims to resources would outweigh those of Alzheimer's patients, or what assurances of actual redistribution would need to be made, this argument nevertheless often seems to exert considerable intuitive pull: There is something unjust, it is said, about committing large amounts of resources to people who are "already gone" while denying help to others in current need.

While it is usually considered a distinct argument, this appeal to justice nevertheless trades on the claims involved in the issues we have already discussed, those of autonomy and mercy. After all, justice in the distribution of resources presupposes that potential claimants to these resources would actually wish to have them or that the receipt of them would actually count as a benefit. If a prospective claimant would not want the resources and they would not be a benefit to him or her, then a distributive scheme allocating resources to this party is unjust if there are other claimants who would want the resources and for whom they would be a benefit. Like the proverbial "dog in the manger," there is no justice in allocating scarce resources to a party who cannot use them; similarly, there is no justice in allocating them to a party who does not want them. Yet given the indeterminate results of the preceding sketches of the issues of choice and mercy, it is by no means clear that Alzheimer's patients "want" the resources that might be allocated to them or that these resources would count as a "benefit."

It is important to note that this is not the same as the "useless eaters" argument advanced by the Nazis as grounds for the destruction of mentally retarded persons and others, though it would have been applied in some of the same cases. The "useless eaters" argument does not assert that the use of resources is not of benefit to the person in question; it asserts that this use of resources is not of benefit to others in the sense that the person in question is "useless" to society. There is no issue in the current question about whether the Alzheimer's patient is "useful" to others, but instead about whether the resources are useful to him or her. Although the two arguments are easily confused, there is in the background of the current discussion about justice in Alzheimer's the assumption that whether or not Alzheimer's patients are "useful" to others or to society in general, society is willing to provide care that is useful to them.

But this then returns us to the problem. Does the Alzheimer's patient want the resources, and are they a benefit to her? Even if claims on her behalf are pressed by a surrogate, can these claims reflect either substituted judgment or any form of best-interests test? Clearly, the more advanced the deteriorative process, the less plausible it is to speak of contemporary choice in wanting resources: The severely demented patient cannot, presumably, understand any other arrangement of things, nor can she conceptualize the distributive schema itself or the allocations it makes to her in competition with others. Nor, presumably, can the severely demented patient in any conscious sense "want" the continuing life that medical treatment and maintenance care make possible, though of course her bodily processes may continue to operate in the normal, life-continuing way; as we said, this person can no longer have any conception of what life is or of the transition from life to death. Of course, she may have had a vigorous conception of all these things prior to the onset of serious disease and may have recorded her wishes in a living will or other document; in this sense, the now-demented person still may "want" access to resources she earlier chose. She can also react favorably to situations she experiences as pleasant and react negatively to those that involve discomfort or pain; in this sense, she can "want" allocations of resources that provide her with, say, foods she prefers, a more comfortable bed, better-fitting clothing (but not more stylish clothing, since appreciating style requires cognitive abilities), and so on. But she can neither conceptualize these wants nor, except by expressions of pleasure or displeasure, articulate them.

Can the severely demented patient benefit from the allocation of resources to her care, including medical treatment, maintenance care, and whatever else is necessry to keep her alive? The answer here is clearly dependent on the argument considered earlier about mercy, and hence we cannot arrive at any clearer answer. Does she benefit from remaining alive, or would she be better off dead? There is quite a lively discussion in the philosophic and economic literature about the value of life, and how one can weigh this against death (Brueckner and Fischer, 1986; Brock, 1986), but it is not a discussion that proves decisive in the present case. Many or most of the features that are usually said to make life worth living are absent in advanced dementia—for example, the possibilities of enjoying human interaction, planning and undertaking projects, serving causes, having religious and aesthetic experience, and perhaps (as Aristotle would identify as the highest good) rational contemplation. With no surviving conceptual skills or even sense of self, it is not clear that continuing life is a continuing good, and hence not clear that allocations that make continuing life possible are really a benefit after all. Nor, however, is it clear that they are not.

What, then, is a fair distribution of resources with respect to people with Alzheimer's? It is not clear that we can even begin to answer this question, because we cannot identify either what Alzheimer's patients want or what would benefit them. Furthermore, we cannot identify wants and benefits either on subjective grounds or on objective, quality-of-life ones: We cannot approximate the severely demented person's point of view, and we cannot assess the quality of her life. Of course, to identify what various claimants want and what would be of benefit to them is not all that is involved in settling distributive issues, since many other matters (for instance, deserts, prior claims, needs for rectification) are involved; but one cannot even get off the ground in justifying a given distributive scheme without knowing whether the various claimants to the resources involved actually want and/or would benefit from them. Discussions of distributive justice uniformly assume that the various competing claimants involved all want and would benefit from the resource in question—that is, that they are all appropriately considered *claimants*—but in the case of Alzheimer's no such thing is clear. Since the amount of resources involved in the issue of

Alzheimer's is immense, the quesiton of justice is an enormous one, and to say that we simply cannot resolve it on adequate philosophical grounds is no trivial matter.

DEVELOPING POLICY CONCERNING EUTHANASIA IN ALZHEIMER'S

Of course, positions on the issue of justice are ultimately expressed in social policy, which puts into practice one or another distributive scheme allocating resources to or away from various claimants or apparent claimants for them. Needless to say, the development of social policy in the matter of allocating resources in Alzheimer's is a matter with such high stakes that it can hardly wait for philosophers to sift through these questions, especially when there is no indication that they will reach a uniform, workable answer. In the absence of firm philosophical justification, then, what form should social policy take in expressing these issues of justice?

To simplify a huge range of possibilities, there are three principal candidates for social policies distributing medical and supportive care in Alzheimer's:

1. do what is possible to maintain and supply medical and supportive treatment for Alzheimer's patients, though without heroics, until the end of their natural lives;
2. practice passive euthanasia on late-stage Alzheimer's patients: provide maintenance and support but not lifesaving medical treatment, and so allow these patients to die when infections or other potential fatal conditions arise; or
3. practice active euthanasia on late-stage Alzheimer's patients.

Current social policy, not at all well defined, wavers between alternatives #1 and #2, though #2 is never termed "euthanasia." It is #3 that raises the question under discussion here. In the absence of firm answers to the questions of choice and mercy, we must still answer the question, Should we, or should we not, practice active euthanasia for Alzheimer's patients? To refuse to address this question is already to answer it, since current social policy prohibits active euthanasia, though permitting passive euthanasia, and to refuse to raise the question is to accept the current answer. It is not clear, however, that this answer is a defensible one. But perhaps there are still other ways of looking at the issue.

THE VIEW DOWN THE SLIPPERY SLOPE

Another, more clearly consequentialist way of approaching the issues in euthanasia in Alzheimer's, or for that matter any proposed social policy, is to take a look down the "slippery slope," that is, to examine the likely highly negative outcomes of introducing the policy. The slippery-slope argument as usually employed against euthanasia predicts the spread of medical killing from a few sympathetic cases, genuinely dictated by the wishes of the patient or the demands of mercy, to more problematic medical cases, then to cases of expensive patients, then to politically undesirable cases, and finally to widespread holocaust. Regardless of whether the advanced Alzheimer's patient wants or would benefit from continuing life, it is argued, active euthanasia ought not be employed, for this would risk the spread of this practice to other persons who both want to remain alive and would benefit by doing so.

Slippery-slope arguments trade on empirical claims about likely consequences, either direct causal results of a certain policy or consequences resulting from other forces affected by the precedents set by a policy. Much of the continuing argumentation about euthanasia involves trading claims about how far the slide would go and how broad the spread of the increasingly intolerable practice would be, and it very often cites catastrophic events such as the Nazi Holocaust as evidence for its claims. When these slippery-slope arguments do so, they generally trade on assumptions about the evil motives of human beings and of physicians in particular, often making reference to the Nazi doctors and their increasing callousness about human experimentation and killing.

It is true that the Nazis' early T4 program began with medical "euthanasia" and that medical staff from this program were later transferred to the extermination camps; but this historical transition does not establish that any practice of euthanasia will always lead to holocaust or that human beings generally or physicians in particular are evil. There are apparent counterexamples: Active euthanasia is practiced in contemporary Holland without evident abuse, and it was also apparently practiced (by recommending the hemlock) in ancient Greece (Battin, 1982, p. 22). However, while the empirical issues can hardly be settled here, it is reasonable to suppose that human beings generally and physicians in particular rapidly respond to incentives of various kinds, especially legal and financial ones.

If active euthanasia in advanced Alzheimer's were legal or legally tolerated in the United States, I think we can well imagine the rapid development of cost-saving social policies that would offer fairly strong incentives for physicians to recommend euthanasia in Alzheimer's, say by reducing reimbursements for treating such persons, by limiting bed space for patients with this condition, or by reconceptualizing the practice as a humane, appropriate course of treatment in this condition.

On the other hand, since any spread of such policies beyond advanced Alzheimer's would be rapidly challenged by other groups whose own interests might be threatened, I see no reason to assume that even if active euthanasia were permitted in some sympathetic cases in advanced Alzheimer's, involuntary euthanasia would inevitably spread to wholesale slaughter of the handicapped, the racially despised, or the politically rejected.

Thus, while I do not think the broad form of slippery-slope argument—which predicts the spread of euthanasia into widespread holocaust—is plausible, at least in the contemporary United States, I can nevertheless imagine the spread of active euthanasia in Alzheimer's from some few cases to a more general policy of comparatively routine use of euthanasia in advanced dementia, and will grant this limited version of the slippery-slope claim here. Routine use of active euthanasia in advanced Alzheimer's might or might not involve solicitation of consent from family members—no doubt it often would, but in the same perfunctory way that consent for no-code orders is now often solicited—but the point is that one can imagine euthanasia as a widespread, medically customary response to severe, irreversible dementia.

Suppose, then, that most or all severely demented, advanced Alzheimer's patients—all million or so—were routinely euthanized, though this practice did not spread to any other category of patient. This is the view down the slippery slope; but the question is how we should assess the view we see. Would this be a bad thing? How are we to answer this question at all? We might try to assess the effects of such a policy on the persons involved, but given the difficulties we have just experienced in considering issues of autonomy and mercy, it is not at all clear that this will be possible to do: We have no way of approximating a subjective assessment and no way of making an objective one either (Nagel, 1986). Nor can we determine whether this widespread practice would be just or unjust. Nevertheless, there is a way of approaching an answer, by looking down the slippery slope in a rather different way.

Doing so appropriates the Rawlsian device of the original position, in which rational self-interest maximizers who are behind the veil of ignorance and thus do not know their own personal characteristics agree to principles that will govern the society of which they are members (Rawls, 1971). However, while Rawls does not discuss health policy and does not use this device for direct policy formation, specific features of the circumstances allow us to adopt it in a rather natural way. This is made possible by the fact that, with respect to the possibility of becoming a patient with Alzheimer's, we are naturally in a kind of "original position" and behind the veil of ignorance: We know the general incidence of severe dementia—about 1 percent between ages 65 to 74, rising to 7 percent between 75 and 84, and to 25 percent for those 85 and over (Office of Technology Assessment, 1987, p. 9)—but as individuals we do not know whether we will be among those affected or unaffected. This provides us with a natural way of considering what principles we would assent to, in seeking to protect our own self-interests, and hence what policies we would be willing to formulate. Thus, rather than speculate about the effects of such a policy on others, we can ask—that is, each of us can ask—whether our own worlds would be better ones for us if, should we become demented, our lives would be protected or would be terminated in euthanasia?

Clearly all the issues we have considered in reflecting on the arguments from autonomy, mercy, and justice reemerge here. However, since the slippery-slope argument is essentially an argument from fear and each potential target of the policy may in principle share this fear, let us look down the slippery slope from the point of view of a single individual who might have such fears. Thus we can ask a more personal form of the question, Would I be more afraid, or less so, in a world that practiced active euthanasia on severely demented Alzheimer's patients? To what sort of policy would I, without knowing into which category I will eventually fall, consent?

Exactly what do I fear, then, in fearing euthanasia, if the slippery-slope prediction comes true and I, like other Alzheimer's patients, may be killed? Assume that I have not previously executed a living will requesting euthanasia, or even that I have no living will indicating any treatment preferences at all. Euthanasia performed on me will be clearly nonvoluntary. This is the scene I can imagine:

Golden Harbor Nursing Home. Morning. The nurses' station in the hallway, then my room. A young doctor, wearing a standard white coat and stethoscope but with steel-rimmed glasses and a slightly disordered crop of thick brown hair, flips quickly through my chart. He extracts a little plastic-coated chart labeled "Functional Criteria in Alzheimer's Disease" from his pocket, checks it, flips through the chart a little further. "I think it's time for Mrs. Battin," he says absently to the nurse, then moves to my room.

"Good morning, Mrs. Battin," he says cheerily, though he already knows I will not respond. "What day is it today?" I tell him a few words, though they are not days of the week. "Who is the President?" I tell him a few more words, though I do not name this fellow Bush, and the doctor makes notes in my chart. He does a variety of other tests, none of which I pass. He or the other doctors like him have done these tests every month for the past half year, and I never show any improvement; now I have failed again. As he goes out I hear him mutter, "Yes, it's time." When the nurse comes in, she is equally cheerful. "So it's time, Mrs. Battin, is it?" She also knows that I do not understand. A phone call will be made to one of my children, explaining the situation and proposing a date; this child will phone the other one, and they will agree.

They will both fly to this city, where the Golden Harbor Nursing Home is; and they will come here to see me for the last time. They do this even though they know I will not recognize them, and have not recognized them for some time. They will try once more to make conversation, though they know it is futile, because they do not know what else to do or how to relate to their mother. They will try to help me remember my husband, though I no longer can, and they will try to elicit even the tiniest fragment of memory. In between, they talk about the house and the arrangements with the lawyer about the estate, though they do not seem to have any particular interest in this—no, they are sad, I see a tear forming in the eyes of one of them, they both grasp my withered old hands, stroke my cheek. They rub, caress my hands and cheek as if they were trying to implant them forever in their own memories. Now they are both crying. After a little while one, then the other, bends over the bed to kiss me. "Goodbye, Mom," each of them finally says, and then they stand and leave, looking back once or twice over their shoulders.

The young doctor is there in the corridor. "Would you like to be with her?" he asks. He notices their own age and the early symptoms of decline: One of them is 57 already, and the other almost 60. One of them wavers a bit, but the other says no. "She wouldn't know we were there anyway," he explains, but the doctor understands why: They are not used to death, and it would be a difficult thing for them to watch. There are a few papers to sign, but that is all; no one objects to the procedure.

The nurse has the syringe already filled for the doctor as he returns to the room, and out of sheer habit she swabs the injection site with alcohol. I say a few more miscellaneous words, and the nurse puts her hand gently on my forehead as the doctor positions the syringe. I feel only a little prick, like so many injections I have had before, and then after that the doctor leans over my chest with his stethoscope to listen to the silence where the heartbeat had been.

So this is how it might go, in an ordinary nursing home, with an ordinary doctor, with an ordinary old lady in the later stages of progressive dementia. If the predictions of the slippery slope are correct, this is how it might go in many nursing homes, all over the country, with all sorts of doctors, with virtually all the 1.5 million patients in the late, irreversible stages of progressive dementia.

And what are my fears, as a likely victim of this spread? Pain? Loss of dignity? Being constricted by involuntary choice? The cursoriness of the visit from my children? Having my life ended without my consent by a physician I don't even know? But of course, I can have experienced none of these things, and indeed my imagined account of these events is entirely misleading: I experienced no pain, nor any loss of dignity; I could not make a choice nor know if my choices were being countervened. I heard the doctor say "it's time," but had no way of understanding what he meant. Although my children's visit was cursory, I did not recognize them as my children. That this doctor was different from the previous one could not have made any difference to me: I could not have known whether I had ever seen him before. I did not know that I had passed or failed any tests, or even that they were tests at all. What was my actual, direct experience in euthanasia? Life as usual until the very end, except for a gentle hand on my forehead and a small needle-prick in my vein. What we fear, in fearing the kind of widespread practice of euthanasia which the slippery slope predicts, are all things we can now imagine but could not then experience; in this sense, our most personal fears are completely unrealistic. This is not the comparison between subjective and objective views of the events contemplated, but between two different forms of subjective view.

What if, on the other hand, there were no euthanasia for severely demented patients, and, as in option #1 above, such patients were provided full maintenance and medical treatment?

Golden Harbor Nursing Home. Morning. Same year as before, then a year later, then sometime during the following year, then at various intervals after that. The young doctor in the corridor, but a different one each time. In the first episode my activities are reassigned to a group for more demented patients, and I now spend the days sitting vacantly at a table with crayons and coloring books in a continuously monitored dayroom; in the second, I am treated for a pneumonia; in the third, I am put in restraints in a day chair; in the fourth, treated for another pneumonia and also decubiti from prolonged sitting; in the fifth, I am spoonfed. Perhaps somewhere in the series I develop paranoid delusions or undergo episodes of random aggressive behavior. By the end of the series, some ten or twelve years later, I cannot communicate at all or walk or get out of bed or feed myself or bathe or control my bladder or bowels. My children have still made a dutiful point of coming to visit me from their respective cities at least once a year, and they still pay the bills, but now they do so with a sense of sullen resignation. The end finally comes with a cardiac arrest, probably about 3 A.M., but it is not noticed until the first nursing round in the morning.

So this is how it might be in an ordinary nursing home, with an ordinary string of doctors, for an ordinary old lady with Alzheimer's. What is there to fear in this scenario? The deterioration I do not notice, since I cannot remember myself as I was nor compare previous stages to this one, nor do I recognize my children at their many visits. But I do experience some new things: I am feverish with infections, I feel the discomfort of the bedsores and, if they are not treated properly, smell their bad odor; I have foods put into my mouth, some of which I like but some I do not; I cannot move my arms out of the restraints on my day chair; I feel the irritation of sitting sometimes for hours in a diaper soiled with urine or feces. If there is any struggle at the end, I, no doubt like many of the other million Alzheimer's patients in the same condition and indeed the rest of the several million who will soon reach this condition, am alone while it happens. But it makes no difference; this nursing home, like most, does not perform CPR.

Is this a better scenario or a worse one than the scenario involving active nonvoluntary euthanasia? Clearly the effects on my children are worse, since they have had no genuine contact with me for years but continue to make their annual visits and to pay the bills; they are no longer sad, but resigned and sullen. Is it better for me? I have been alive for all these years; but I can think of no compelling reason to say I would not have been better off dead, that is, without any experience at all. Of course, there have been positive experiences—a shaft of sunlight warming my cheek through the slats of the venetian blind in my window, well-meaning hugs now and then from an indefatigable nursing staff or from visitors I do not know—but there are also the diapers, the restraints, the bedsores, and the espisodes of illness and infection which I cannot understand but for which I am treated. If my claim to care under distributive scarcity rests on the assumption that I want this continuing life or that it is a benefit to me, is my claim really secure?

But what about the apparent compromise position, #2? This is the position that represents an increasingly pervasive policy today: to take advantage of intercurrent infections or illnesses and, by refraining from providing treatment, let the patient die. This is the compromise position favoring passive euthanasia (though it is rarely called that), which rejects both indefinite extension of life and active termination. What would it be like, and could I fear it? The scene at Golden Harbor will be the same as before, except that various young doctors will not order treatment for various infections or illnesses, and I will survive a few of these, though with difficulty, until finally one of them kills me. My children will be summoned hastily, or perhaps after the fact, but will have had no general sense of where in the overall downhill course of my progressive dementia my death might occur, whether a few years earlier or perhaps a lot of years later. My sensory experiences, though shorter, will have been in one way worse than the second series above—I will have endured at least one or perhaps several episodes of illness without treatment, or with only whatever symptomatic control is possible consistent with letting the disease take its course. The difference between alternative #3, active euthanasia, and this one, #2, passive euthanasia, is that in the former the doctor killed me; in the latter, it is a disease that does the killing. When the doctor killed me, my only experience was a gentle hand and a tiny needle-prick; in alternative #2, I am "allowed to die," and this necessarily occurs only at the conclusion of a period in which I am mortally ill.

Why then should I fear the slippery slope, or let it count as a persuasive argument against euthanasia? Even if we grant that the spread that this argument predicts would actually occur and some 1.1 million currently institutionalized Alzheimer's patients would be medically killed, as well as the rest of the several million whose disease eventually progresses and in addition all new cases developing, it is not clear that *from the point of view of each of them* this would be a bad thing. Figures in the millions, of course, recall the appalling butchery of the Holocaust, but that killing viewed from the points of view of each of those victims was a catastrophically bad thing. After all, the victims of the Holocaust wanted to stay alive, in the sense discussed earlier, and would clearly have benefited from doing so. But the victims of Alzheimer's are different. After all, their points of view will be exactly like my own, accurately and not unrealistically imagined, if I should develop Alzheimer's—a point of view without a sense of self, without cognitive capacities for comparing one's past and present circumstances, without memory, without the ability to understand or predict death, and with only the capacity for current sensation. As a rational self-interest maximizer who does not yet know whether I will or will not develop Alzheimer's, can I fear euthanasia, if this is what my future may hold? Clearly the answer is no.

Of course, there may be aspects of euthanasia I could fear—for instance, that the doctor would be hasty or irresponsible in conducting the tests of functional capacity, that the nurse would be rough, that the nursing home would be callous in contacting my children. To be sure, medical personnel and institutions can be hasty, rough, and callous in all sorts of situations, but there is no special incentive for acting in this way in the case of euthanasia; on the contrary, given special legal protections, the presence of witnesses, and so on, one might expect incentives to run the other way. If I have no reason to fear euthanasia in principle and no reason to think that in practice it would be cruelly conducted, there seems to be no basis for responding to the slippery-slope argument at all. Generalizing thus from my own imagined single case behind my current veil of ignorance to that of severely demented persons generally, it looks, on the contrary, as though alternative #3, a world of routine active euthanasia, rather than passive euthanasia or continuing treatment, would better protect my self-interests; hence it is the policy to which I would agree.

DEVELOPING SOCIAL POLICY

Philosophical reflection seems to produce no compelling argument against euthanasia in advanced Alzheimer's and no sound reason why we should fear it. Should we then, as a matter of social policy, practice nonvoluntary active euthanasia on advanced Alzheimer's patients, developing a set of guidelines for functional status which would serve to determine the appropriate timing—guidelines that the physician could, like the young doctor in the Golden Harbor Nursing Home, carry around in his pocket on a little laminated card? If this seems a disturbing suggestion, reopening all the fears the slippery slope points to, it is important to be clear about what the problem is.

The problem in developing policy, I think, arises from the difference in the perceptions the public is likely to have of this issue and what philosophic reflection produces. Ordinary—that is, precritical, nonreflective, nonphilosophical—perceptions of the prospect of nonvoluntary euthanasia are likely to take the form in which our little scenarios here have been described; it is the way most of us see this issue most of the time. We tend to see the issue from the point of view of a conscious, self-aware person (ourselves now) capable of remembering and comparing circumstances and engaging in human relationships, not from the point of view of those persons actually affected by the practice, namely those persons who are severely demented (ourselves in a possible future). In reflecting on the nature of euthanasia and the possibility of the slippery slope, we do not readily assume the perspective of the persons most directly affected, but rather our own *current* view. This is why the little imagined descriptions presented earlier are so misleading: They presuppose the wrong point of view. They are fictions in the fullest sense, even though they purport to describe a possible future. The imaginary account of euthanasia in the Golden

Harbor Nursing Home involves a narrated personal experience—the doctor enters *my* room, looks at *my* chart, asks *me* questions that provide a diagnostic test, listens to the garbled answers *I* tell him, prepares to inject the euthanaticum into *my* vein. This little story is narrated in a temporal sequence as seen from an individual point of view, that of the self to whom it would happen; but of course this is a misleading description of the experience of a severely demented person. This is not what will happen to me, not because it will not happen, but because if I am severely demented, it cannot happen to *me*.

But while imaginary narratives of this sort—developed as a way of employing a natural version of the Rawlsian device for selecting principles and at the same time as a way of looking down the slippery slope—are misleading in one way, they are enormously useful in another. For they also provide a way of foreseeing what problems certain social policies might cause. In this sense, fiction serves as forecast. If it is correct that, as ordinary human beings, not philosophers, we are more likely to view the prospect of widespread involuntary euthanasia from our own current perspective than from the perspective of ourselves in the future, a policy permitting involuntary euthanasia of millions of advanced Alzheimer's victims might well produce considerable anxiety, even anguish, for most of us, depending on how these stories are interpreted. Of course, it is anxiety to persons *before*, though not after, they contract Alzheimer's; but it is still a kind of anxiety to be considered in developing social policy. Indeed, anxiety before, rather than after, developing advanced Alzheimer's is the only kind of anxiety which can be experienced, insofar as it is anxiety about what will happen in the future to oneself and hence presupposes the cognitive capacity both to anticipate the future and to entertain a conception of oneself.

Furthermore, philosophic reflection can also produce anxiety of another sort for possible future Alzheimer's patients: the anxiety of recognizing that the prevailing policies #1 and #2, favoring continuing treatment or allowing to die, are really much less defensible than they may seem. The anxiety results from knowing that these policies are unlikely to change, and that if one does develop Alzheimer's, these indefensible policies will govern how one is treated. Furthermore, this anxiety is compounded by knowing that once one is in the circumstances in question, one can no longer do anything to change them and can no longer protect oneself from being governed by them, say by executing a directive stipulating exactly how one wishes to be treated.

Thus, in thinking about social policy and on what basis it is to be formulated, we see we are faced with two kinds of anxiety: that produced by ordinary, unreflective attitudes about euthanasia in Alzheimer's, and that resulting from considered, philosophical reflection at odds with the ordinary view. These are two forms of subjective view, as I've mentioned earlier, not a subjective and an objective one, and neither has clear pride of place. The real question here is whether social policy ought to be formulated on the basis of one rather than the other, and if so, which one—for they will produce very different policies indeed. Basing policy on the ordinary view will be a vote for the status quo; basing it on the considered, philosophical view will support policies endorsing nonvoluntary active euthanasia in advanced dementia. Permitting active euthanasia only in conjunction with an antecedently executed living will or personal directive requesting it is probably the best policy compromise, since this appears to protect against unreflective fears of nonvoluntary euthanasia but protects those who make antecedent choices on more philosophical grounds. Yet even this compromise policy provides little guarantee that, as we formulate social policies that will determine our own possible futures whether or not we contract Alzheimer's, we will be able to keep considerations based on fiction distinct from those based on philosophy.

ACKNOWLEDGMENTS

The author thanks Virgil Aldrich, Leslie Francis, and Brooke Hopkins for discussion of this chapter.

REFERENCES

Battin, M.P. (1982). *Ethical Issues in Suicide.* New York: Prentice-Hall.

Battin, M.P. (1987). Euthanasia. In D. VanDeveer and T. Regan, eds., *Health Care Ethics: An Introduction*, pp. 58–97. Philadelphia: Temple University Press.

Brock, D.W. (1986). The value of prolonging human life. *Philosophical Studies*, 50:401–428.

Brueckner, A.L., and Fischer, J.M. (1986). Why is death bad? *Philosophical Studies*, 50:213–221.

Dworkin, R. (1986). Autonomy and the demented self. *Milbank Quarterly*, 64(Supplement 2):4–16.

Nagel, T. (1986). *The View from Nowhere.* New York: Oxford University Press.

Office of Technology Assessment, Congress of the United States. (1987). *Losing a Million Minds: Confronting the Tragedy of Alzheimer's Disease and Other Dementias.* Washington, D.C.: U.S. Government Printing Office.

Rawls, J. (1971). *A Theory of Justice.* Cambridge: Harvard University Press.

PART III. Caring for People with Dementia: Justice and Public Policy

10

DEMENTIA
AND APPROPRIATE CARE:
ALLOCATING
SCARCE RESOURCES

Daniel Callahan

The dementias pose a special problem for our health care system, and in particular they put to a severe test common attitudes about allocation priorities in the care of elderly people. While younger people are afflicted, the dementias (particularly Alzheimer's disease) are characteristically diseases of older persons, increasing in prevalence with increase in age. Data suggesting that more than 50 percent of those beyond the age of 85 may be afflicted dramatically underscore that point (U.S. Department of Health and Human Services, 1989, p. 1). Like the old age of which they are a part, the dementias are at present incurable, presenting in their pathological course the classic symptoms of a slow, chronic, degenerative disease. Not only do they bring down their victims in a cruel and implacable way, but they also pose heavy demands on family members and caregivers. Their victims require a great deal of personal care, and care always overshadowed by the inevitability of decline and death.

The dementias deserve the highest priority in health care for elderly people. This is not because they have a fatal outcome. A lethal disease in old age is not necessarily a tragic outcome, but an inherent part of the human condition. It is instead because of the unique capacity of the dementias to rob old age of dignity and quality, often bringing down at the same time spouses and other family members.

THE BIAS AGAINST CARING

It will not be easy to give the dementias a high priority in actual policy, however much media attention and public interest they have gained in recent years. The peculiar allocation problem we face with the dementias is that the features they display tend to bring out the worst in the American health care system, and the demands they place on the system—especially for personal care and social services—are just those we have most commonly resisted. Our society can get enthusiastic about finding a scientific cure for a fatal disease. It is far less zealous about providing the sustaining services necessary to help its victims endure their illnesses until such a cure is found. Its zeal to help family members and others to cope with the social and psychological burdens of caring for the ill is even fainter.

The fact that there is no medical treatment available for the dementias, whether for cure or relief of symptoms, also places them outside the preferred mainstream of American health care. Diseases of slow decline, presenting few acute phases and unresponsive to available technologies, are almost guaranteed a second-class citizenship in our health care system. That's not what we are good at, not what we have designed the system to manage, and not what gives us our greatest therapeutic thrills.

Can this bias be changed? That is, can we change the direction of a system that is heavily oriented toward cure rather than care, a system that will handsomely finance lifesaving dialysis treatment for the elderly, even for those in otherwise poor condition, or coronary bypass surgery for octogenarians with only a statistically short life expectancy thereafter, but cannot find the money to provide the victims of Alzheimer's the less dramatic long-term and home care services they need, much less support and respite for their caregivers?

At present the odds for that kind of change are not great. It will require a revolution in our thinking and our practices. We have created a health care system addicted to life extension and fully prepared to pursue that goal with high-technology medicine. As a result, the medical education system, the hospitals, and the reigning therapeutic philosophy are powerfully oriented in that direction; that, in turn, shapes practices, attitudes, and expectations.

This bias can be seen in the care of both the young and the old. In the case of the young, we will spend an enormous amount of money on a child with low birth weight in a neonatal unit, but then frequently leave the child's parents bereft of adequate resources for continuing follow-up care and treatment once out of the hospital (Nolan, 1987). In the case of the old, there is a powerful trend toward applying to them the benefits of high-technology medicine, ordinarily by taking procedures originally developed for younger persons and applying them to those who are older. It is no accident, for instance, that a study undertaken at the Mayo Clinic found a fivefold increase in surgery for those over the age of 90 in the last ten years, or that heart and liver transplants have been extended strikingly to those in their 60s and even 70s, or that the fastest-growing group of those on dialysis are over age 65 (Hosking et al., 1989; de Lissovoy, 1988; Health Care Financing Administration, 1987). Treatments of that therapeutic, surgical, and technological kind are well supported by Medicare; no one has to "spend down" their economic assets to qualify for them. The same is not true for the social services and long-term care more characteristically required by those suffering from Alzheimer's. They typically fall under the much more poorly financed Medicaid program (responsible for long-term and home care for the elderly), not Medicare, and thus that is where the greatest need lies (Office of Technology Assessment, 1987, pp. 415–443).

SETTING LIMITS ON HEALTH CARE EXPENDITURES

It can of course be argued that this kind of imbalance in available entitlement programs is simply wrong, scandalously so, and that the answer is just to increase resources to meet the needs of dementia victims without in any way restricting resources for all the other needs of the elderly, especially those where we have already made a commitment to acute-care medicine and maximum life extension. We could, in other words, just buy our way out of the problem by spending more money.

That response can no longer have the public appeal it once did, and perhaps rightly so. In the United States we already spend a larger proportion of our gross national product (GNP) on health care, and more per capita, than any other nation—but with no better health outcome than most other developed nations. While there is widespread dissatisfaction with the costs of health care, there is little willingness to pay higher taxes to have a better, more equitable system (Melville and Dolbe, 1988). The public and legislative resistance to ever higher taxes may not quickly pass. Moreover, even if we could find more money, and achieve that other great nostrum—more efficiency, less waste in the system—there are other severely pressing societal needs, other than health, requiring large public and private investment, most notably education, housing, and basic economic development.

There is increasingly little reason to continually expand resources for health care when so many other sectors are suffering even worse deprivations. This means, then, that we will have to develop a philosophy of health care in general, and for the elderly in particular, which can better help us learn to live within some prudent boundaries. By "prudent" I mean recognizing that we cannot let health care command a disproportionate share of total national resources, or health care for the elderly a disproportionate share of total health resources.

Since we are faced with an enormous increase in the number and proportion of the elderly in coming decades, and with the likelihood of a no less steady increase in expensive technological capabilities of extending their lives, that will be a difficult task. Central to that task will be the need to find a better balance in expenditures between aggressive curative medicine and the more patient, caring medicine needed to cope with chronic conditions such as Alzheimer's.

A NEW PHILOSOPHY OF HEALTH CARE FOR ELDERLY PEOPLE

That kind of a balance will only be likely if we can develop a more coherent, rounded philosophy of health care for the elderly. We require a philosophy that recognizes that the elderly need not an aggressive search for a longer life as an age group, but the avoidance of a premature death and the living of a decent quality of life within that boundary. Our present implicit philosophy—as evidenced by our practices, insurance coverage, and entitlement programs—is heavily biased toward curative medicine.

One problem here is obvious: There is no end to the possibility of spending money to combat the inevitable biological decline and inevitable death that are inherent in aging. Unless curbed, therefore, a curative bias will effectively consume a disproportionate share of resources as it pushes forward the frontiers of life extension, a frontier that is in the nature of the case open and endless. It is disproportionate precisely because it seems to make it almost certain politically that the kinds of nursing, custodial, familial, and social service needs that the dementias generate will be the comparative losers—needs that are, I believe, no less important for the overall welfare of the elderly. The large and increasing amount of money going to the present Medicare program, woefully deficient in its coverage of all but acute-care medicine, effectively blocks other needed programs. The chances are slight that a good long-term care program will gain support in the face of so-far uncontrolled acute-care costs under the present Medicare programs. Only by curbing our appetite for ever improved, ever more expensive high-technology medicine will we be in a position to right the imbalance between curing and caring.

That is also an appetite that effectively works to rob old age of meaning, though this has yet to be sufficiently noticed. Its implicit premise is that the only meaningful old age is one that places the highest priority on averting death, not on marshaling our resources to help make of old age a time of completion and enrichment.

Let me propose a speculative hypothesis. It is probably no accident that the campaign against ageism is roughly coincidental in time historically with a Medicare program oriented toward cure rather than care. It is a campaign that, for all of its many virtues in trying to uproot demeaning stereotypes about the elderly, may be inadvertently robbing old age of the possibility of any deep common meaning.

How could that be happening? By its insistent emphasis on the individuality and heterogeneity of the elderly rather than on their common and general features, the anti-ageism movement (at least in much popular if not academic understanding) has minimized just those features of aging which have always been needed to make sense of old age as a part of the life cycle and in the biographical life of the individual. Those features include a recognition that the elderly must pass social leadership to the young, that the social significance of old age lies in its capacity for generativity and for a transmission of the culture to a younger age group, and that old age is a time to collect and complete the self, not to pretend that meaning can only be had in more life. The very idea of a reciprocal set of obligations between young and old, a trait of all decent cultures, assumes that the elderly are as identifiable an age group as the young.

An anti-ageist philosophy, worried mainly about prejudice toward the old, seems at times to have too little room for the other side of the coin: finding a way to think about what it means to grow old as part of our human condition, a general problem and one that can never properly be grasped by a reductionistic individualism stressing the heterogeneity of the old (Butler, 1975; Neugarten, 1982). When that kind of individualism is combined with a no less individualistic medicine—invariably oriented toward cure because among other things it reduces our dependence on one another—the result can be oppressive. It is a medicine reluctant to accept our common fate, which is aging, decline, and death.

Anti-ageism and high-technology medicine make ideal partners, each confirming the bias of the other, the former intent on minimizing the general features of aging, the latter bent on endlessly patching up individual human bodies pulled down by their mortality.

A philosophy of medicine and aging oriented toward caring and quality of life, by contrast, can better situate the individuality of the person within a context of social interdependence and a more prudent acceptance of mortality. It is of course the essence of Alzheimer's that death will follow deterioration, that its victims require the care of others in the absence of cure, and that it most clearly and unmistakably points to the limitations of our well-established glorification of that medicine that would banish our illness and delay our dying, not try to help us better accept and live with them. Alzheimer's disease, in short, is an embarrassment to contemporary medicine. It has everything scientific medicine seems, at least implicitly, to want to eliminate: mortality, mutual human neediness, and the demand for the most personal, and demanding, self-sacrifice on the part of family members. For that is precisely what a full cure of the disease would accomplish. Failing to get that, medicine is left at sea, forced to settle for second best, something it does not do well.

I am certain there will be some who will continue to argue that we can have it all: that we can seek more and better—indeed, unlimited technological and curative medicine for the elderly—as well as provide better long-term and home care. But the historical record in this country speaks strongly against that likelihood, and the actuality of the present Medicare system, already financially expansive and increasingly demanding, speaks all the more against it as a practical possibility. No less important, the very premise of the emphasis on cure works against decent long-term and home care as well, for it is a premise that says caring is inferior to curing, a second-best choice, and that acceptance of limits to decline and mortality is inferior to efforts to transcend them. This premise worked well enough in an earlier era, when the infectious diseases were gradually being eliminated. It has been a great mistake to assume that premise will remain equally true in the face of the degenerative diseases associated with aging.

CHANGING OUR PRIORITIES

We have yet to take the full measure of what may be an unavoidable outcome of the effort to extend life—that of the generation of increased morbidity and chronic illness. The fastest-growing age group in this country is that of persons over 85, and it appears to be no accident that the increase in prevalence of Alzheimer's is a consequence of that growth. Here we see one of the most vexing, unpalatable features of the effort to modernize mortality by constantly extending curative medicine. We have been saved from death by infectious diseases in childhood, only to be exposed to death by cancer, heart disease, and stroke in our later years, and if we can get past them long enough, we are then ripe for Alzheimer's. It is a necessary, though not sufficient, basis for Alzheimer's that we age long enough to get it; and the more we age, the more likely it becomes. All the more reason, then, to wonder if the emphasis on cure is an unmixed blessing. Not only does it set us up to require more care when the cure fails (as ultimately all cures must fail), but it also seems to guarantee that we risk using a disproportional share of our resources for that quest before we get there—not a nice outcome.

I have been proposing so far that a health care philosophy for the elderly oriented toward a better balance between curative and caring medicine would most serve the needs of dementia victims. Yet such a philosophy must be set within the health care system as a whole, one responsive to the needs of all age groups. My own belief is that the most sensible set of priorities for the health care system would place care (by which I mean both nursing care and broad social service provisions), not cure, at the top of the list, and all the more so in an era of chronic disease and diseases of aging not readily amenable to cure. Thereafter as priorities should come general public health measures such as immunization, health promotion and disease prevention, basic biomedical research, and good primary and low-technology emergency care. At the very bottom of my priority list would come high-technology medicine oriented toward individual care.

I am not here in any way suggesting the elimination of such medicine; we can afford a great deal of it. I am only suggesting that it should have a lower priority in the future, that is, we should not pursue and disseminate it with unbounded zeal until we have taken care of other, more pressing needs. Of course quite the opposite of the priorities I am suggesting has been the pattern in the United States—and that is exactly why the dementias have not fared well.

A similar set of priorities would be appropriate for the elderly as well, though here it would also be necessary to specify more fully some reasonable goals of the health care system in providing for them. My own preference would be for an approach that aimed to avert a premature death, which sought for each person a full life cycle—which can be had amply if never totally by the late 70s or early 80s—and which thereafter worked primarily to provide as high a quality of life as possible, not necessarily a longer life. Whether or not the theory of a compression of morbidity hypothesized by James Fries ever proves itself as a fact, it does provide a potent heuristic basis for policy: that of aiming to reduce morbidity and disability within a decently long life span, but not aiming to lengthen that life span (Fries, 1989).

By every standard I have so far suggested, then, Alzheimer's would receive a high priority, indeed the very highest. While it is eventually a fatal disease, its most striking feature is its effect on the quality of life of its victims. That fact, plus the obvious reality that it is so far incurable, gives it a primary claim on caring, intensified all the more by the demands it makes on family members. Research on the disease should have a high priority as well, ideally producing a cure that would be amenable to a public health approach, such as immunization, rather than an expensive therapeutic approach. The latter has, unfortunately, so far been the case with AIDS, amenable only to a life-extending, not lifesaving, drug treatment of an expensive kind—that is, AZT

(Scitovsky, 1989). It is of course possible that something similar could happen with Alzheimer's, and that would surely pose a great crisis. No doubt our society would come up with the money, but probably at the cost of neglecting the health needs of other groups of patients, young and old. In any case, we would be wise not to bet on a cure or an ameliorative drug for Alzheimer's in the foreseeable future, much less drag our feet on greatly improving long-term and home care as well as social services out of a hope that a cure will be found.

In the face of scarcity, however, would it be justifiable to shift money from the present Medicare system, with its emphasis on curative medicine, to an improvement in the kind of long-term and home care services needed by dementia victims? I believe it may be necessary two or three decades from now to set an age limit on government reimbursement of expensive life-extending treatments for those elderly who have already lived full lives (Callahan, 1987). Yet we are nowhere near that point of necessity now, and we have not put in place the long-term and home care policies that are indispensable prerequisites. It could, however, be justifiable to limit to less than full reimbursement coverage and benefits for acute-care treatments in the near future in order to (a) begin reducing the commercial and medical incentives to continue devising new ways to expensively extend life expectancy in the elderly, and (b) help make available more funds for long-term and home care. Unhappily, we do not have in place the kinds of planning and policy mechanisms to make such a trade-off possible or morally safe. We desperately need such mechanisms.

The balance between care and cure as an emphasis in the health care system is not yet necessarily a zero sum game. But we may be near that situation, both because of voter resistance to higher taxes and because of the doubtful wisdom of increasing general health care expenditures in the face of other societal demands even more pressing. As the economist Uwe Reinhardt noted, "Total taxes in this country at all levels of government have, in effect, fluctuated very narrowly around a fixed level of 33 percent of GNP since 1970, in spite of an aging population and a growing underclass of poverty-stricken children. . . . Given this relatively small, fixed public budget, every dollar the American public health sector must spend on health care must come at the expense of other public expenditures—including spending on the nation's public infrastructure and on education" (Reinhardt, 1989, p. 18).

To that observation I would add: In the face of pressures to hold down health care cost increases, any money spent on acute-care medicine is money withheld from long-term and home care. The fact that acute-care medicine gained the initial high ground, prestige, and medical priority in the 1960s and 1970s—and then had that priority established in federal entitlement programs—only adds to the difficulty of dislodging it. Yet that is exactly what must be done, however difficult it will probably be. Those reformers who continue to hold out for an expansion of both acute-care medicine and a medicine of caring and social support have increasingly little reason to be hopeful. While there has been increased talk of some form of universal health insurance, as well as improved long-term care, it is difficult to find any congressional observers, much less members, who believe it is likely in the near future. The failure in early 1990 of the Pepper Commission—established by Congress to develop plans for improved health care for the poor and for a revitalized long-term care program—to come up with any proposals at all for the estimated \$63 billion in additional funds necessary to pay for those improvements was not a happy augury for the future.

SCARCE RESOURCES AND DEMENTIA PATIENTS

I have so far focused on questions of the broad allocation of resources at the policy level. How might we best think about resource allocation at the clinical level, particularly when an Alzheimer's victim is faced with an acute, life-threatening event? This is a delicate issue for a number of reasons. First, by virtue of the Alzheimer's, the patient is already caught in a terminal illness, even if it is one that is gradual. Is it reasonable and best for the patient to save him or her from the acute incident when we know that will simply extend the dying from Alzheimer's? Second, even if we decide that it is for the patient's good that he or she should be saved, can we justify a large expenditure from a familial or societal perspective? One might answer such a question "of course we can," and that would certainly be my initial instinct. But if "large" becomes "damagingly large"—that is, threatening the basic welfare of others—that should make us pause. It is not as if we are helping the patient recover from the underlying Alzheimer's; indeed, our acute-care intervention only allows the Alzheimer's to continue all the longer. Even if the cost of saving a patient's life is relatively low in individual cases, the aggregate costs of doing so for the estimated 2.53 million cases at present, or the 5 million estimated by 2040, are surely heavy (U.S. Department of Health and Human Services, 1989, p. 1).

Let me put to one side here the question of what is to be done when the patient had earlier left clear instructions about what he or she desired if caught in a condition of this kind. In that case, the patient's wishes should be followed. But there will be many other circumstances where prior instructions—a living will or a durable power of attorney document—will not exist. It will then become the obligation of the patient's family and physician to determine the morally proper course of action. My own conviction is that, as a general rule, questions of resource allocation should not enter into treatment decisions of individual patients. Instead, once in the health care system, those patients should receive whatever is appropriate for them as individuals. It is within the system itself that the limits should be set, binding physicians in their clinical decisions. Any limitation of services or care should, that is, be established by general policy, not determined by individual doctors dealing with individual patients at the bedside. The only exception that seems justifiable would be that of an emergency triage situation, such as an immediate shortage of intensive care unit (ICU) beds.

But would a dementia, in and of itself, qualify as a good reason to establish a general policy of limitation of acute-care, life-extending medicine? To be more specific, would it be reasonable, say, to have a rule denying Alzheimer's patients access to an ICU, or to dialysis? No. Such a flat rule would not be justifiable. An obvious objection is that the disease would not necessarily be far advanced in all cases; some patients on the borderline could have some years to live, not all of them severely demented. Still another objection is that the acute-care medicine might be necessary as part of decent caring medicine—for instance, to relieve pain and suffering rather than to extend life.

Nonetheless, even if it would be a mistake to invariably deny acute-care, life-extending medicine to someone who is demented, we can ask a narrower question. Would it be morally defensible as a general, though not invariably binding, rule to withhold acute-care, life-extending medicine from severely demented patients—that is, to say that unless there are strong and clearly specifiable reasons to override the rule, life-extending acute-care medicine should not be deployed in advanced dementia cases? I believe it would be, but because of the condition, not primarily the age, of the patient. The obvious and ordinary justification for the use of acute-care medicine is to restore a patient to, or maintain a person in, a state of health sufficient to maintain the integral personhood of the patient, not simply the bodily organs of a person. In the case of severe dementia, that personhood has been severely compromised, its potential gradually dying (as is also, in the case of Alzheimer's, the patient's body).

It is thus hard to see why there would be an obligation to work aggressively by means of the most advanced medical treatments to extend life under those circumstances, to forestall death from a relievable acute condition in order to allow more time for a gradual decline and death from the dementia. What is the benefit to the patient? There is no obvious good answer to this question. There are no discernible human benefits in a gradual demise through dementia, none at all. Why, then, would we want to avert the possibility of a more rapid death if this entailed no greater suffering for the patient? Why is a later death from dementia (or some other acute illness that might emerge) humanly preferable to an earlier death from another condition? Put another way, if a patient is in the grips of a downward trajectory with an inevitably lethal outcome preceded by gradual distintegration of all characteristically human potentialities, why would we want to aggressively intervene to save the patient from a possible shortening of that trajectory by the fortuitous appearance of another lethal condition? I can find no good answer to that question.

While age as such has not entered into the way I have formulated the moral problems, advanced age should serve to relieve us all the more of any lingering doubts we might have about our culpability in not initiating acute-care treatment. A person of advanced old age is in the grips of a condition of aging which is ordinary biological evidence of the close relationship between aging and death, sooner or later in the life cycle of the individual. We can try, as many do, to distinguish between becoming old and becoming sick. At some time or other, however, the two conditions will coincide in the life of the elderly person. Decline and death from Alzheimer's at an advanced age would seem an obvious illustration of that reality (even if we can imagine finding a cure for Alzheimer's someday).

Let me bring this discussion to an end by trying to join the approach I suggested for the policy issue of allocation of resources to the demented elderly, and that of the clinical treatment of individual dementia patients. Because we do not now have a cure for the dementias, especially Alzheimer's, a policy bias in favor of a greater emphasis on caring medicine in old age, rather than acute-care, life-extending medicine, would be especially helpful to its victims and their families. They are the losers in a system now biased toward curative medicine. At the same time, a bias (though not a flat rule) against acute-care medicine for individual dementia patients, especially those with well-advanced cases, would seem the morally appropriate response to their inevitable decline and death; no good purpose would be served by that kind of medicine in those cases. Comfort and palliation would, of course, always be appropriate, no matter what the condition of the patient; they are standing requirements of good patient care and medical morality.

What we need, then, is an entitlement policy that better supports and serves those whom we cannot cure. Accompanying it should be a treatment policy that once again recognizes that death is not necessarily a medical failure (as was the case in the long history of medicine prior to the scientific era of relatively recent decades), but to be welcomed in those cases where more physical life contributes nothing to human dignity and personhood.

REFERENCES

Butler, R.N. (1975). *Why Survive? Being Old in America*. New York: Harper and Row.

Callahan, D. (1987). *Setting Limits: Medical Goals in an Aging Society*. New York: Simon and Schuster.

de Lissovoy, G. (1988). Medicare and heart transplants: will lightning strike twice? *Health Affairs*, 7(Fall):61–72.

Fries, J.F. (1989). The compression of morbidity: near or far? *Milbank Quarterly*, 67(2):208–232.

Health Care Financing Administration. (1987). *Special Report: Findings from the National Kidney Dialysis and Kidney Transplantation Study*. Baltimore, Md.: U.S. Department of Health and Human Services.

Hosking, M.P., Warner, M.A., Lobdell, C.M., Offord, K.P., and Melton, L.J., III. (1989). Outcomes of surgery in patients 90 years of age and older. *Journal of the American Medical Association*, 261(13):1909–1915.

Melville, K., and Doble, J. (1988). *The Public's Perspective on Social Welfare Reform*. New York: Public Agenda Foundation.

Neugarten, B. (1982). Policy for the 1980s: age or need entitlement? In B. Neugarten, ed., *Age or Need? Public Policies for Older People*, pp. 19–32. Beverly Hills, Calif.: Sage Publications.

Nolan, K. (1987). Imperiled newborns. *Hastings Center Report*, 17(6):25–30.

Office of Technology Assessment, Congress of the United States. (1987). *Losing a Million Minds: Confronting the Tragedy of Alzheimer's Disease and Other Dementias*. Washington, D.C.: U.S. Government Printing Office.

Reinhardt, U. (1989). Health care spending and American competitiveness. *Health Affairs*, 8(4):5–21.

Scitovsky, A.A. (1989). Studying the cost of HIV-related illnesses: reflections on the moving target. *Milbank Quarterly*, 67(2):318–344.

U.S. Department of Health and Human Services. (1989). *Report of the Advisory Panel on Alzheimer's Disease: 1988–1989*. Washington, D.C.: U.S. Department of Health and Human Services.

11

THE POLITICS OF DEVELOPING
APPROPRIATE CARE
FOR DEMENTIA

Robert H. Binstock

Thomas H. Murray

As the twentieth century draws to a close, the goal of achieving humane and appropriate care for victims of dementia, as well as for other patients who need long-term care for chronic illnesses and disabilities, is becoming widely shared in the United States. Opinion polls indicate that a substantial majority of Americans—in all adult age groups—fear the financial, familial, psychological, and social consequences of long-term care and favor the general principle of expanding government insurance to reimburse long-term care services adequately (McConnell, 1990).

The central ingredient for achieving appropriate long-term care, as indicated in chapter 1, is massive financing for it. A number of policy options for such expanded financing are currently being explored and debated (see Ball, 1989; Rivlin and Wiener, 1988; OMB Watch, 1990; Wiener, 1990). Estimates of the amount of additional resources needed to fund these options range as high as $50 billion a year.

Among those who share the goal of better care there is substantial disagreement regarding the most appropriate and effective strategies to secure the tens of billions of dollars needed to finance it, particularly through governmental policies. One point of view is that reform and adequate financing of long-term care is only feasible in the context of policies that set limits on the use of health care resources for medical interventions that "cure" patients who are of an advanced age. Adherents to this view argue that resources saved by such limits would be subsequently reallocated to long-term care. In effect, they see an ample expansion of resources for long-term care produced as a by-product of "rationing" acute care. But such a perspective is neither dictated by the economics of health care in the United States nor based on a realistic assessment of the politics of public resource allocation. Indeed, framing policy issues from this perspective may retard, rather than accelerate, a substantial expansion of public long-term care resources.

An alternative view, presented in this chapter, argues that adequate long-term care is most likely to be realized through a direct and explicit national policy that specifies new tax revenues to expand substantially the public resources available for such care. Political support for such a policy will need to be developed through extensive grass-roots consideration of fundamental issues regarding the role of government in financing long-term care. Such issues include: Why should moderately well-off and wealthy persons be protected by government from having to spend their income and assets on long-term health and social care? Which citizens might be taxed to preserve the income and assets—and ultimately the legacies—of others? Do we want to have our government undertake more active steps than at present to preserve economic status inequalities from generation to generation?

These are but a sampling of the basic issues that we need to confront and resolve through extended public discourse if a genuinely adequate level of financial and political support for long-term care is to develop in our society. Without a conscious dialogue on such issues, any new public policies on long-term care are likely to suffer the same fate as the short-lived Medicare Catastrophic Coverage Act of 1988, repealed in 1989—a policy developed by public elites in Washington, without any grass-roots understanding, feedback, and popular political support.

Widespread debate on such issues, moreover, may also help us to clarify some of the broader issues of distributive justice which are embedded in strategies for reforming the availability and provision of health care in the United States. Is there a morally relevant difference between one group—be it the aged, the demented, the poor—and any other which justifies unequal treatment in the provision of acute or long-term health care? Should different standards of equity be applied to the health care arena than those applied to other spheres of activity in our society? As political philosopher Michael Walzer (1983) argued, in a democratic society the answers to such questions are appropriately and most likely to be resolved through a process of widely shared decision-making that is attentive to both the particular nature of the goods and services being distributed and the society's most deeply held values.

COULD RATIONING ACUTE CARE FOR OLDER PEOPLE
FUND LONG-TERM CARE?

Some philosophers, biomedical ethicists, and policy analysts argue that the best approach for funding an expansion of long-term care is by rationing some of the acute care—especially technology-intensive, and expensive, health care—which is currently provided to older persons (e.g., Daniels, 1988; Lamm, 1989; Menzel, 1990; Veatch, 1990–91). In the present political environment, saturated with public rhetoric expressing concerns about the rates of growth in federal budget deficits and health care expenditures, they assume that some new form of health care rationing is both inevitable and imminent in the United States. And in this context they contend that the most just and feasible source of funds to finance appropriate long-term care is the savings that could be reaped by denying lifesaving care to older persons.

Perhaps the most eloquent and publicly prominent spokesperson for this general point of view is Daniel Callahan. His thoughts on these matters, as exemplified in the preceding chapter of this volume, have been widely disseminated in the past few years through two books (Callahan, 1987; 1990a), a number of journal articles (e.g., Callahan, 1988; 1989; 1990b), and public appearances. His argument is that adequate funding of long-term care should only be obtained by reallocating funds that are customarily expended on acute care for elderly people. He urges us to "recognize that we cannot do everything, that it will be impossible to burn our economic candle at both ends, trying to provide basic social and nursing services while at the same time chasing endless technological progress to extend life. The price of having the former is to radically curtail the latter" (Callahan, 1989, p. 365).

This *radical curtailment* that Callahan espouses, as spelled out in his seminal book on this theme (1987), would be brought about by using "age as a specific criterion for the allocation and limitation of health care" (p. 23) by denying life-extending health care—as a matter of public policy—to persons who are in their "late 70s or early 80s" and/ or have "lived out a natural life span" (1987, p. 171). What is a "natural life span"? According to Callahan, the natural life span is a matter of biography rather than biology. He uses chronological age as an arbitrary marker to designate when, from a biographical standpoint, the individual should have reached the end of a "natural life," and be viewing life retrospectively rather than prospectively.

Callahan's proposal to deny lifesaving health care on the basis of old age, and similar proposals of other commentators, break new ground in philosophies about health care in America. To be sure, health care in the United States has long been rationed on the bases of social class and ability to pay (Churchill, 1987; Hiatt, 1987), the immediate availability of resources (Blank, 1988), and the individual conditions and characteristics of patients. But an explicit policy that would deny health care to people solely on the basis of their membership in an age group—or in any other demographic category such as race, ethnicity, or religion—would be a substantial, indeed, a drastic, departure from existing philosophies and practices.

As drastic as such proposals are, no persuasive arguments have been made to justify the notion that rationing the health care of elderly people is an essential step for funding long-term care, or even that any new form of rationing is necessary at all (see Binstock and Post, 1991; Etzioni, 1991). The economic arguments for old-age–based rationing rest on unwarranted assumptions and are poorly developed. The pleasant policy scenarios in which the funds saved from rationing would be reallocated to fund long-term care, or any other worthy items on a "wish list," are politically and financially unrealistic.

IS FURTHER RATIONING OF HEALTH CARE INEVITABLE?

A basic premise underlying old-age–based rationing proposals is that explicit health care rationing is inevitable and imminent in the United States (see Lamm, 1989; Aaron and Schwartz, 1990) and that we are bringing about some sort of economic crisis by spending nearly 12 percent of our gross national product (GNP) on health care (Lazenby and Letsch, 1990). But proponents of rationing may have misdirected our attention to other issues. The first poses the question, Whose health care must be rationed? As Callahan (1989) framed the issue, "One way or another, we will have to ration health care" (p. 353). Another issue, as articulated by Callahan: "How does the use of age as a standard for limiting health care compare with other unpleasant methods of limitation? We need to pit the methods of rationing against each other, not against the ideal world in which we all wished we live" (pp. 356–357). Yet it is far from self-evident that drastic new rationing schemes are necessary at all.

Is there an economic crisis, current or impending, engendered by health care expenditures? Advocates of health care cost containment warn that we cannot economically sustain increasing health care expenditures. Why not? What are the inevitable dire consequences that would ensue for our nation (as opposed to specific health care payers and providers) if health care expenditures continue to grow?

It is not at all clear, for example, that escalating health care costs hurt the global position of the U.S. economy. Joseph S. Nye, Jr. (1990), debunking "The Misleading Metaphor of Decline," points out that the U.S. share of the world gross product (WGP) has held constant at 23 percent since the mid-1970s. And Alfred Balk (1990), author of a recent book entitled *The Myth of the American Eclipse*, presents an impressive list of indicators—such as America's share of world exports, control of high-technology industries, productivity per worker, global investments, and predicted long-term shares of WGP—which suggests that popular laments regarding the decline of the American economy are nonsense.

In theory, of course, it can be argued that the American economy might have an even stronger position in the world if it were not for the proportion of our wealth spent on health care costs. A fashionable expression of this perspective is the complaint made by some corporate executives and health care policy analysts that the competitiveness of American business firms is hurt by the fact that about 10 percent of payroll expenses in our medium-sized and large industries goes to employee health insurance (McNerny, 1990). But these health insurance fringe benefits merely substitute for either larger wages and salaries or other types of fringe benefits that would be used as alternative components in the total package of employee compensation (see Uchitelle, 1991). As health economist Uwe Reinhardt (1990, p. 174) noted, "It does not make sense to pick out one of these components and blame it for problems American business faces in pricing its products."

In short, it is far from self-evident that U.S. health care expenditures are unsustainable. Eli Ginsberg summarized the situation very well:

> There is nothing inherently bad about the expenditure of $620 billion on health care services by a $5 trillion economy. Nor is there any reason a $6 to $7 trillion economy should not spend $1 trillion or even more for its health care. The nub of the issue is whether the U.S. economy will grow in the decades ahead at an average rate of 1.5% per annum or at a rate of 3%. At 1.5%, increasing health care costs could preempt most of the increment in gross national product; at a 3% growth rate, which translates into an addition of $150 billion, the nation will be able to cover a rising health care bill and still have considerable remaining for other socially desirable uses such as increased expenditures for education, housing, and infrastructure. High-tech medicine is not the villain and its restraint is not a preferred strategy; slow economic growth is the challenge to meet and overcome. (Ginsberg, 1990, p. 1822)

Health care cost containment is not an end in itself, and is not mandated by any "iron law" of economics. As many observers have pointed out (e.g., Schwartz and Aaron, 1985), there is no inherent reason why 12 percent, 13 percent or more of our GNP cannot be expended on health care. The proportion of our national wealth which we can and ought to invest in health care is not a technical issue of economics, but a value judgment to be resolved through politics.

There may be a sense of crisis about costs, but health care resources, in general, are certainly not growing scarcer. Rather, they are expanding (Waldo et al., 1986; Letsch et al., 1988; Health Care Financing Administration, 1990). The problem is not scarcity but an unwillingness and/or an incapacity of our political system to allocate them through some other means than economic and social stratification. Reinhardt explained the situation very clearly: "If the American public, and the politicians who represent it, really cared about the nation's indigent, they ought to be able to exploit the emerging surplus of health care resources to the advantage of the poor" (Reinhardt, 1986, p. 29).

WOULD FUNDS SAVED BY RATIONING BE USED FOR LONG-TERM CARE?

Although setting limits to the health care of older persons is not dictated by economics, it clearly is a political and moral choice preferred by Callahan and other proponents of old-age–based rationing. They justify their views with arguments that the funds saved by denying efforts at lifesaving cures for elderly people might be reallocated to long-term care and palliation—in nursing homes, hospices, and residential settings—for those older persons afflicted with chronic disabilities and illnesses, such as an estimated 3.5 million persons with Alzheimer's disease. Even as older persons become socialized to the notion that they will be denied lifesaving health care, it is argued, they can look forward to the months and years still available to them as ones that can be finished out relatively free of pain and avoidable suffering (see Callahan, 1987, p. 135).

There are no particular reasons, however, why one health care objective has to be achieved at the expense of another, except within the context of a specific health care budget that is inadequate to meet all the health care needs of the population that it serves. Such trade-offs do take place in the context of health care systems that have fixed budgets, such as the British National Health Service, where some health care procedures are rationed to enable health care districts to stay within their budgets (see Aaron and Schwartz, 1984). Similarly, some managed health care entities in the United States, such as health maintenance organizations financed by annual per capita fees, also make trade-offs motivated by budgetary concerns. And the state of Oregon has recently made a political decision to put a ceiling on its annual Medicaid budget. It has developed a list that gives priority rankings to medical procedures—applied to patients described by age categories and gender, as well as health care needs—and has hired actuaries to estimate just how far down this priority listing the annual Medicaid budget will be able to fund treatments of Medicaid patients (Egan, 1990; Fox and Leichter, 1991; Kitzhaber, 1990–91). Oregon now seeks from the federal government a procedural waiver that would enable the state to deny Medicaid reimbursement for health care procedures that rank below the actuarially determined cutoff point (Brown, 1991).

Neither Medicare nor the overall American health care system operates within a predetermined budget. Little in American political experience suggests that funds saved from financing one cause are likely to go to other, preferred and predesignated causes. In fact, recent experiences suggest—and emphatically underscore—just the opposite. The "freed-up" resources that we thought might be available from the post–Cold War peace dividend (see Beatty, 1990) were more than exceeded by expenditures that were on no one's "wish list," such as the savings and loan bailout. Did any of us think when Secretary of Defense Richard Cheney canceled contracts for the further development of the A-12 navy attack plane in 1991 that the more than $2 billion saved through this decision would be used to fund program expansions in prenatal care, immunization of children, or Head Start?

The notion that funds conserved by denying health care to older people would be earmarked through some sort of rationalized central planning process and reallocated for long-term care is politically unrealistic. New federal programs get financed through explicit policy initiatives to deal with them, not through decisions to eliminate existing commitments. For example, when President Bush proposed to reallocate $58 million from existing community health programs in order to finance a campaign against infant mortality in ten cities in early 1991 (Pear, 1991a), he was sharply rejected by members of Congress in both parties (Pear, 1991b, 1991c). In contrast, each of the half dozen major bills introduced in Congress in the past few years to provide expanded federal funds for long-term care has been premised on the notion that new taxes—not reallocated funds from existing forms of health care—will and should be used to finance the expanded coverage.

HOW MUCH LONG-TERM CARE COULD BE FINANCED BY RATIONING?

What if we were to develop a societal consensus—as urged by Callahan—that lifesaving care should be denied, categorically, to persons in their late 70s and older? What sorts of financial "savings" might be achieved through such rationing? If the resources conserved by setting limits to expensive acute care for older persons were applied to the long-term care of victims of dementia and other chronic diseases and disabling conditions, how much of the estimated need for such care would they meet? How would such savings compare in magnitude with the savings that might be achieved through other, less morally troublesome measures directed toward expenditures in health care or other arenas?

Proponents of old-age–based rationing have not identified the magnitude of savings which might be achieved through their proposals. But, for illustrative purposes, it is possible to construct a relevant example.

About 28 percent of annual Medicare expenditures is on those Medicare insurees who die within a year, but only 3 percent of these decedents are relatively high-cost cases (Lubitz and Prihoda, 1984). Suppose we were to deny care to prospective high-cost decedents (although, clinically, it is rarely possible to make highly reliable prospective distinctions between high-cost survivors and decedents).

Even if it were ethically and morally palatable to implement a policy that denied treatment to such high-cost Medicare patients, and thereby eliminate "wasteful" health care, the dollars saved would hardly begin to fund the estimated annual cost of adequate long-term care. High-cost Medicare decedents annually account for 3.5 percent of Medicare expenditures (Lubitz and Prihoda, 1984). In 1990, when Medicare expenditures totaled $111 billion, a policy that denied treatment to these patients would have saved about $3.9 billion.

This potential savings of $3.9 billion would only fund a small fraction of the costs of an expanded public long-term care program, which have been estimated to be as much as $50 billion in the first year (OMB Watch, 1990). Moreover, if there is some sort of crisis in health care costs, saving such an amount would have a negligible effect on the overall situation in a year when national health care costs totaled $666 billion (Reischauer, 1991).

It is easy enough to recognize that $3.9 billion in savings from the so-called "wastes" on health care for older persons is dwarfed by the savings that could be achieved by setting limits on other types of expenditures that, from a societal point of view or as matters of personal values, can be labeled as undesirable or frivolous—federal subsidies for tobacco; luxury items such as furs, jewelry, and yachts; and even the health care of cats and dogs. Orthopedic and heart surgery on household pets can cost from $1,500 to $4,000. In 1987, Americans spent nearly $6 billion on veterinary services, including CAT scans and pacemaker implants (Nordheimer, 1990).

But even if it were economically imperative that human health care costs be reduced, how does the total that might be saved by rationing the care of older persons compare with other areas of potential savings in American health care expenditures? Just the bureaucratic aspects of our health care system in themselves seem to provide a promising arena for saving unnecessary expenditures. A few examples should be sufficient to illustrate that the resources that might be saved by eliminating "fat" in our health care system far outweigh the $3.9 billion expended on high-cost Medicare decedents in a twelve-month period, in attempts to save those patients' lives.

The proportion of U.S. health care spending consumed by administration is at least 117 percent higher than in Canada; if health care administration in the United States had been as efficient as in Canada in 1987, the savings to our system would have ranged from $69 billion to $83 billion (Woolhandler and Himmelstein, 1991). The Health Insurance Association of America estimated that about $60 billion in fraudulent or abusive private and governmental insurance claims were paid in 1989 (Rosenthal, 1990). According to Joseph Califano, Jr. (1991), former secretary of the Department of Health, Education, and Welfare, more than $25 billion a year could be saved by standardizing, simplifying, and electronically processing reimbursement claims and audit procedures. Medicare pays about $600 million to $1 billion a year in reimbursement claims that have already been paid by private insurers or should have been (Pear, 1990). Medicaid spends more than $500 million a year more for pharmaceuticals than would be necessary if that program required drug manufacturers to give it price discounts similar to those provided other bulk purchasers such as hospitals, health maintenance organizations, and the departments of Defense and Veterans Affairs (Freudenheim, 1991; Pear, 1991d).

THE POLITICS OF FUNDING LONG-TERM CARE

Effective and humane provision of long-term care is too important, for most of us, to rest on an illusion that it will be financed as a by-product of policies that set limits to lifesaving care for older persons and the comparatively small savings that might thereby be achieved. Indeed, if we were to become preoccupied with old-age–based rationing as the means of achieving appropriate long-term care, we would probably delay rather than facilitate long-term care reform. As Callahan noted in calling for many years of discussion on his proposal: "Nothing other than a long-extended public debate over many years is likely to suffice. . . . A proposal to limit health care for the aged will be seen as coercive. . . . Only a full-scale change in habits, thinking, and attitudes would work to make it morally and socially possible" (Callahan, 1987, p. 158).

In the meantime the tens of billions of dollars needed to fund a substantial expansion of public long-term care insurance are far more likely to be raised through legislation that generates new governmental revenues to fund the policy, as has been the case with other major initiatives for older persons such as Social Security and Medicare (see Cohen, 1985a, 1985b; Derthick, 1979; Iglehart, 1989; Light, 1985). For those of us who would like to facilitate such an expansion, what feasible strategies are available to us?

THE LEGACY OF THE CATASTROPHIC COVERAGE ACT

Although long-term care is now on the agenda of Congress and may stay there in the immediate future, it is not at all clear that a bill will be enacted for some years to come. As suggested earlier, the lessons that members of Congress learned from the birth and rapid demise of the Medicare Catastrophic Coverage Act of 1988 have made them more aware than they were of the high financial costs of insuring long-term care and, especially, the political risks involved in levying new taxes to pay for it (Atkins, 1990). There are also some positive lessons from the Catastrophic experience, however, which can be applied by advocates who seek the enactment of a major long-term care program.

The Catastrophic Act was the first major expansion of benefits to older persons in sixteen years. It provided insurance coverage for economically catastrophic hospital and physician bills, for outpatient prescription drugs, and for some elements of long-term care (Medicare, 1988). The estimated costs of these new benefits (and administration of them) totaled about $31 billion for fiscal years 1989 through 1993.

From all accounts the White House and congressional leaders self-consciously determined that the new benefits would be "self-financed"—that is, paid for wholly by elderly persons themselves through Medicare Part A and Part B premiums—rather than funded through Federal Insurance Contribution Act payroll taxes or general revenues (Iglehart, 1989). Congress planned to raise 37 percent of the new financing by adding $4 a month to the premiums paid by all Medicare Part B enrollees. The remaining 63 percent of the needed revenues was to be raised through a "supplemental" premium, or Part A tax, to be paid by middle- and higher-income older persons— approximately 40 percent of participants—on the basis of their federal income tax liability. In 1989, each Medicare enrollee was to pay $22.50 a year for every $150 of income tax liability, up to a limit of $800 per individual and $1,600 per couple.

The development of this legislation was due to the initiatives of public officials in the White House, Congress, and the bureaucracy who were focused on their own agendas for social and economic policy (see Iglehart, 1989). Dr. Otis Bowen, secretary of the Department of Health and Human Services when the legislation was proposed and enacted, had favored catastrophic-illness coverage through Medicare for many years. Such coverage became a Reagan-administration legislative proposal when Bowen responded to the president's 1986 State of the Union directive that the Department of Health and Human Services develop options to protect all Americans against the economic consequences of serious illness (Bowen, 1987).

During the subsequent period of nearly two years before the bill became law, neither Congress nor the so-called aging-advocacy groups (such as the 35-million-member American Association of Retired Persons) floated "trial balloons" or lofted "political footballs" to enable some 30 million older Americans to understand what sorts of benefits they would receive through the new Catastrophic Act, and who would pay for them. No feedback was effectively obtained regarding the millions of older persons who already had private insurance coverage for some of the major benefits being offered (see Crystal, 1990), and for the outrage that middle-income Medicare participants would feel regarding the amount of surtax they would be expected to pay. Consequently, no base of popular support was built for catastrophic coverage, and no legislative refinements were made to tailor the new benefits more carefully and make the surtax scale more tolerable.

When the proposal finally did become a law, there was no popular constituency supporting it. But there was distinct opposition to it, symbolized by some militant older persons who expressed their displeasure by climbing on top of the automobile of Congressman Dan Rostenkowski, chairman of the House Ways and Means Committee, when he visited his home district in Illinois. Nationwide protest from a relatively small, unrepresentative group of comparatively well-off older persons—upset by having to pay a new progressively scaled surtax for benefits they thought they already had—cowed Congress into repealing the legislation in 1989 (see Tauke, 1990). As Representative "Pete" Stark, an author of the repealed Catastrophic Act, put it, "We are being stampeded by a small group to deny benefits to everyone else." And Rostenkowski added, "Because we in this Congress can't take the heat from the wealthy few, all principles are abandoned" (Tolchin, 1989a).

Why did Congress reverse itself so quickly and easily? One simple explanation, as suggested by Stark and Rostenkowski, is that politicians characteristically distance themselves from any matters that are reviled by even small vocal proportions of their constituencies. A concomitant explanation is that the Catastrophic Act was not developed with any grass-roots understanding and support for its content.

Opponents, those who had to pay the most taxes and who perceived that they already had the coverage to be provided through the new law, were a small numerical minority (Findlay, 1989; Tolchin, 1988, 1989a, 1989b). But they were dispersed throughout every congressional district. When they protested vociferously against the act, Congress received no evidence of countervailing popular support for the bill (despite the fact that it had been endorsed by the Washington-based lobbyists for the American Association of Retired Persons). Indeed, it appeared that many older persons were under the impression that the bill was going to cover primarily the catastrophic costs of long-term care, rather than catastrophically expensive hospital and physician bills stemming from extended acute care.

APPLYING THE LESSONS TO LONG-TERM CARE POLITICS

What political lessons can be learned from the Catastrophic catastrophe? How might they be applied to the campaign for expanding public long-term care insurance through federal legislation?

One lesson may be that, in the contemporary political context, the traditional elitist "top-down" approach to social legislation, exemplified in the Catastrophic Act, needs to be inverted. "Bottom-up" support for public long-term care insurance will have to be genuinely sought from the grass roots, with desires and demands articulated actively in virtually every congressional district.

A second lesson is that the nature of what is demanded—its details and consequences—should be fairly well worked out and comprehended at the grass-roots level, so that constituents as well as Congress and bureaucrats understand the legislation's implications.

Favorable sentiment has crystallized around the general principle of expanded coverage. But many complex ideological issues are masked by the broad label "public long-term care insurance," and such issues have just begun to surface in public debate (e.g., Eckholm, 1990; Tolchin, 1990). Although a number of different technical approaches to financing and determining eligibility for expanded public long-term care insurance have been set forth (see Spence and Hanley, 1990), they are too esoteric to serve in mobilizing broad political support.

Widespread public debate on underlying values will be required if constituents are to understand the implications of any legislation that is to be enacted. Otherwise, even if enacted, such legislation could quickly be repealed as was the poorly understood Catastrophic Act. Vague sloganeering for long-term care insurance will not be sufficient.

Serious debate on this topic will have to start with the fact that the United States already has public long-term care insurance in the form of Medicaid, for nursing homes; that is, any older person who is sufficiently impoverished to be unable to pay for long-term care out of income and assets becomes eligible for Medicaid reimbursement of services. If a patient has a spouse, he or she is protected by law from impoverishment (Medicare, 1988). Because home care services reimbursed by Medicaid do not usually include all of the continuum that is necessary in a home setting, the Medicaid-financed patient usually ends up as a nursing home resident. So part of the long-term care agenda is public insurance that can provide a genuine choice of home care for poor elderly patients for whom it will suffice.

Most of the current interest in additional public insurance, however, is apparently generated by the possibility of *becoming* poor through "spending down" assets on long-term care. There is a distinct middle-class fear—both economic and psychological—of using savings and selling a home to finance one's own health care. This anxiety reflects a widespread desire to protect inheritances, as well as the psychological intertwining of personal self-esteem with one's material worth and independence.

Yet research findings are beginning to show that the incidence and prevalence of the spend-down phenomenon may be grossly overestimated. One recent nationwide study (Liu et al., 1990), for instance, provides persuasive evidence that only about 10 percent of patients discharged from nursing homes were initially admitted as private pay patients and then subsequently spent down their income and assets to the point of becoming Medicaid patients (see also Burwell et al., 1989; Liu and Manton, 1989). This contradicts a common assumption, previously relied on in research and policy-analysis literature (Branch et al., 1988; Burwell et al.), that 50 percent or more of Medicaid-reimbursed nursing home patients enter the institutions as private pay patients and subsequently spend down until they are poor.

By the same token, it appears that we cannot assume that most nursing home patients who are reimbursed by Medicaid became eligible for that program by spending down until they were poor. Research conducted in 1988 and 1989 by the Office of Inspector General (OIG) of the U.S. Department of Health and Human Services provides substantial and convincing nationwide evidence that the practices of sheltering and transferring financial assets to preserve them while becoming eligible for Medicaid is widespread. For example, the OIG found that:

> People initially denied but subsequently approved for Medicaid nursing home benefits in Washington state for 1 year possessed $27.5 million in assets at the time of their denial. These assets had to be disposed of before they could qualify for assistance. Over 80% of the assets had been sheltered:

59% were transferred to a spouse, 11% were retained as exempt. Only 8% were consumed for long-term care. The remainder was of uncertain disposition. (Moses, 1990, p. 23)

In short, it appears that many Medicaid patients—with the assistance of legal counsel—have become adept at what one lawyer terms "Avoiding the Medicaid Trap: How to Beat the Catastrophic Cost of Nursing Homes" (Budish, 1989–90). They are able to take advantage of a policy for the poor without being poor. They can preserve their estates and, perhaps, pass them on as legacies, while having government pay for their long-term care.

As implied by these research findings, there are many fundamental issues that we need to confront and resolve if we are to achieve an effective, enduring program of expanded public long-term care insurance. Among these issues are:

- If we can devise effective laws for protecting the spouse of a long-term care patient from impoverishment, why shouldn't people spend their assets and income on their health care? Why should government foot the bill?

- Why should it be government's responsibility to preserve estates? So they can be inherited?

- Should government take a more active role than at present in preserving economic status inequalities, from generation to generation? On what basis should some persons be taxed to preserve the inheritances of others?

- Should the taxing power of government be used to preserve the psychological sense of self-esteem which for so many persons is bound up in their accumulated assets—their material worth?

- Should any specific age or measures of economic worth be used to determine eligibility, or should public funds be available for long-term care patients of all ages and income statuses?

These are some of the basic political issues that must inevitably surface in one form or another if expanded national long-term care insurance is to become a serious legislative proposition. They need to be aired through debate and resolved with widespread understanding. And the responses need to be crystallized fairly well and then conveyed back to Washington in a fashion that indicates widespread constituent support. As the experience of the Catastrophic Act suggests, politically satisfactory answers to such questions will not be worked out well in Washington—either on Capitol Hill or in the bureaucracy.

There are many positive responses to such issues—responses that could provide a strong foundation for a universal long-term care insurance program in the United States. At the very least, substantial debate would make it apparent to most Americans that long-term care, traditionally overshadowed by acute care in public discussions and allocations for health care in our society, is an important part of our contemporary health care scene. Long-term care accounts for about 10 percent of annual health care expenditures (Lazenby and Letsch, 1990). And the odds of any one of us needing long-term care are rather high. Persons who are now 65 years of age have a 43 percent chance of entering a nursing home at some time before they die. Of those who do enter, 55 percent will use nursing homes for a total of at least one year in their lifetime, and 21 percent will have total lifetime stays of five or more years (Kemper and Murtaugh, 1991).

Thorough public discussion of the fundamental value issues that bear on long-term care policies may also lead us to broader ethical and moral perspectives that will enable us to view the health care arena in a more equitable light than we have to date. Perhaps we will see that there are no inherent reasons for making distinctions between age groups, for separating the relatively poor from the relatively wealthy, or for treating long-term care as any less important than acute, life saving care.

Walzer (1983) has pointed out that notions of justice throughout history have varied not only among cultures and political systems, but also among distinct spheres of activities and relationships within any given culture or political system. Nothing requires us to devise or accept separate spheres of justice within health care. Widespread and thoughtful consideration of the fundamental issues that underlie long-term care reform may well lead us, finally, to delineate the health care arena as a sphere of justice within which no distinctions are made among Americans on the basis of their demographic, economic, and social characteristics.

REFERENCES

Aaron, H.J., and Schwartz, W.B. (1984). *The Painful Prescription: Rationing Hospital Care*. Washington, D.C.: Brookings Institution.

Aaron, H.J., and Schwartz, W.B. (1990). Rationing health care: the choice before us. *Science*, *247*:418–422.

Atkins, G.L. (1990). The politics of financing long-term care. *Generations*, *14*(2):19–22.

Balk, A. (1990). America is no. 1. it'll stay no. 1. *New York Times* (July 3):All.

Ball, R.M. (1989). *Because We're All in This Together: The Case for a National Long-Term Care Insurance Policy*. Washington, D.C.: Families USA Foundation.

Beatty, J. (1990). A post–Cold War budget. *Atlantic Monthly, 256*(2):74–82.

Binstock, R.H., and Post, S.G., eds. (1991). *Too Old for Health Care? Controversies in Medicine, Law, Economics, and Ethics*. Baltimore, Md.: Johns Hopkins University Press.

Blank, R.H. (1988). *Rationing Medicine*. New York: Columbia University Press.

Bowen, O.R. (1987). Coverage for catastrophic care. *Human Development News* (May):1, 6.

Branch, L.G., Friedman, D., Cohen, M., Smith, N., and Sokolovsky, E. (1988). Impoverishing the elderly: a case study of the financial risk of spenddown among Massachusetts elderly people. *Gerontologist, 28*:648–652.

Brown, L.D. (1991). The national politics of Oregon's rationing plan. *Health Affairs, 10*(2):28–51.

Budish, A. (1989–90). *Avoiding the Medicaid Trap: How to Beat the Catastrophic Cost of Nursing Homes*. New York: Henry Holt and Co.

Burwell, B., Adams, E., and Meiners, M. (1989). *Spend-down of Assets prior to Medicaid Eligibility among Nursing Home Recipients in Michigan*. Washington, D.C.: SysteMetrics/McGraw-Hill, for the Health Care Financing Administration.

Califano, J.A., Jr. (1991). More health care for less money. *New York Times* (May 14):A15.

Callahan, D. (1987). *Setting Limits: Medical Goals in an Aging Society*. New York: Simon and Schuster.

Callahan, D. (1988). Vital distinctions, mortal questions: debating euthanasia and health care costs. *Commonweal* (July 15):397–404.

Callahan, D. (1989). Rationing health care: will it be necessary? can it be done without age or disability discrimination? *Issues in Law and Medicine, 5*(3):353–366.

Callahan, D. (1990a). *What Kind of Life? The Limits of Medical Progress*. New York: Simon and Schuster.

Callahan, D. (1990b). Rationing medical progress: the way to affordable health care. *New England Journal of Medicine, 332*:1810–1813.

Churchill, L.R. (1987). *Rationing Health Care in America: Perceptions and Principles of Justice*. Notre Dame, Ind.: University of Notre Dame Press.

Cohen, W.J. (1985a). Securing Social Security. *New Leader, 66*:5–8.

Cohen, W.J. (1985b). Reflections on the enactment of Medicare and Medicaid. *Health Care Financing Review, Annual Supplement*:3–11.

Crystal, S. (1990). Health economics, old-age politics, and the Catastrophic Medicare debate. *Journal of Gerontological Social Work, 15*(3/4):21–31.

Daniels, N. (1988). *Am I My Parents' Keeper? An Essay on Justice between the Young and the Old*. New York: Oxford University Press.

Derthick, M. (1979). *Policymaking for Social Security*. Washington, D.C.: Brookings Institution.

Eckholm, E. (1990). Haunting issue for U.S.: caring for the elderly ill. *New York Times* (March 27):1.

Egan, T. (1990). Oregon lists illnesses by priority to see who gets medical care. *New York Times* (May 3):1.

Etzioni, A. (1991). Health care rationing: a critical evaluation. *Health Affairs,* *10*(2):88–95.

Findlay, S. (1989). The short life of catastrophic care. *U.S. News and World Report* (December 11):72–73.

Fox, D.M., and Leichter, H.M. (1991). Rationing care in Oregon: the new accountability. *Health affairs, 10*(2):7–27.

Freudenheim, M. (1991). Pressure grows for curbs on prices of prescription drugs. *New York Times* (May 11):1.

Ginsberg, E. (1990). High-tech medicine and rising health care costs. *Journal of the American Medical Association, 263*(13):1820–1822.

Health Care Financing Administration, Office of National Cost Estimates. (1990). National health expenditures, 1988. *Health Care Financing Review, 11*(4):1–41.

Hiatt, H.H. (1987). *America's Health in the Balance: Choice or Change?* New York: Harper and Row.

Iglehart, J.K. (1989). Medicare's new benefits: catastrophic health insurance. *New England Journal of Medicine, 320:*329–336.

Kemper, P., and Murtaugh, C.M. (1991). Lifetime use of nursing home care. *New England Journal of Medicine, 324:*595–600.

Kitzhaber, J. (1990–91). A healthier approach to health care. *Issues in Science and Technology, 7*(2):59–65.

Lamm, R.D. (1989). Columbus and Copernicus: new wine in old wineskins. *Mount Sinai Journal of Medicine, 56*(1):1–10.

Lazenby, H.C., and Letsch, S.W. (1990). National health expenditures, 1989. *Health Care Financing Review, 12*(2):1–26.

Letsch, S.W., Levit, K.R., and Waldo, D.R. (1988). National health expenditures, 1987. *Health Care Financing Review, 10*(2):109–122.

Light, P. (1985). *Artful Work: The Politics of Social Security Reform.* New York: Random House.

Liu, K., Doty, P., and Manton, K. (1990). Medicaid spenddown in nursing homes. *Gerontologist, 30:*7–15.

Liu, K., and Manton, K. (1989). The effect of nursing home use on Medicaid eligibility. *Gerontologist, 29:*59–66.

Lubitz, J., and Prihoda, R. (1984). The use and costs of Medicare services in the last two years of life. *Health Care Financing Review, 5*(31):117–131.

McConnell, S. (1990). Who cares about long-term care? *Generations, 14*(2): 15–18.

McNerny, W.J. (1990). A macroeconomic case for cost containment. *Health Affairs, 9*(1):172–174.

Medicare. (1988). *Catastrophic Coverage Act of 1988, Title III, Section 303.*

Menzel, P.T. (1990). *Strong Medicine: The Ethical Rationing of Health Care.* New York: Oxford University Press.

Moses, S.A. (1990). The fallacy of impoverishment. *Gerontologist, 30:*21–25.

Nordheimer, J. (1990). High-tech medicine at high-rise costs is keeping pets fit. *New York Times* (September 17):1.

Nye, J.S., Jr. (1990). The misleading metaphor of decline. *Atlantic Monthly,* *265*(3):86–94.

OMB Watch. (1990). *Long-term Care Policy: Where Are We Going?* Boston: Gerontology Institute, University of Massachusetts at Boston.

Pear, R. (1990). U.S. would force private insurer to pay claim before Medicare. *New York Times* (December 21):1.

Pear, R. (1991a). Bush plan to fight infant deaths would use money going to poor. *New York Times* (February 7):1.

Pear, R. (1991b). Bush's infant care proposal draws fire in both parties. *New York Times* (March 6):A11.

Pear, R. (1991c). Spurning Bush, Congress provides new money to fight infant deaths. *New York Times* (March 26):1.

Pear, R. (1991d). Medicaid is denied discounted drugs despite new law. *New York Times* (February 18):1.

Reinhardt, U. (1986). Letter of June 9, 1986, to Arnold S. Relman. *Health Affairs*, 5(2):28–31.

Reinhardt, U. (1990). Health care woes of American business: Reinhardt response. *Health Affairs*, 9(1):174–177.

Reischauer, R.D. Statement of Robert D. Reischauer, Director, Congressional Budget Office, before the Committee on Ways and Means, U.S. House of Representatives (October 9, 1991), mimeo.

Rivlin, A.M., and Winer, J.M. (1988). *Caring for the Disabled Elderly: Who Will Pay?* Washington, D.C.: Brookings Institution.

Rosenthal, E. (1990). Health insurers say rising fraud is costing them tens of billions. *New York Times* (July 5):1.

Schwartz, W.B., and Aaron, H.J. (1985). Health care costs: the social tradeoffs. *Issues in Science and Technology*, 1(2):39–46.

Spence, D.A., and Hanley, R.J. (1990). Public insurance options for financing long-term care. *Generations*, 14(2):28–31.

Tauke, T. (1990). The slow demise of the Medicare Catastrophic Coverage Act. *Aging Network News* (January):7.

Tolchin, M. (1988). Health insurance plan provokes outcry over costs. *New York Times* (November 2):1.

Tolchin, M. (1989a). House acts to kill '88 Medicare plan of extra benefits. *New York Times* (October 5):1.

Tolchin, M. (1989b). How the new Medicare law fell on hard times in a hurry. *New York Times* (October 9):1.

Tolchin, M. (1990). Paying for long-term care: the struggle for lawmakers. *New York Times* (March 29):1.

Uchitelle, L. (1991). Insurance linked to jobs: system showing its age. *New York Times* (May 1):1.

Veatch, R.M. (1990–91). An egalitarian argument for rationing. *Aging Today*, 11(6):9, 11.

Waldo, D., Levit, K., and Lazenby, H. (1986). National health expenditures, 1985. *Health Care Financing Review*, 8(1):L1–21.

Walzer, M. (1983). *Spheres of Justice*. New York: Basic Books.

Wiener, J.M., ed. (1990). *Long-Term Care Financing*. *Generations*, 14(2).

Woolhandler, S., and Himmelstein, D.U. (1991). The deteriorating administrative efficiency of the U.S. health care system. *New England Journal of Medicine*, 324:1253–1258.

12

ALZHEIMER'S DISEASE: CURRENT POLICY INITIATIVES

Gene D. Cohen

The simple dictionary definition of *policy*—a principle, a plan, or a course of action—masks the complexities of its practical application in the area of Alzheimer's disease (AD). Policy-making varies with the level of activity—public or clinical. Of course, public and clinical policy not only may be consistent or homogeneous but also may have heterogeneous influences, such as federal government versus state government views, or administrative versus legislative perspectives at any level of government. Clinical policy, too, is subject to varied orientations, such as those concerned with rehabilitation and cure rather than chronic care (Kane, 1986). To a large extent, the discussion to follow will focus on current public policy.

PERSPECTIVES INFLUENCING POLICY

What one expects with aging influences what policies one considers for older adults. Consider, for example, the views of Shakespeare, in *As You Like It*, and Cicero, in *De Senectute*, which contrast the expectations of growing old as illnesses of later life:

> Last scene of all.
> That ends this strange eventful history
> In second childishness and mere oblivion,
> Sans teeth, sans eyes, sans taste, sans everything.

Intelligence, and reflection, and judgment, reside in old men, and if there had been none of them, no states could exist at all.

Consider what a perspective that views the inevitable concomitant of aging as being "sans mind" could do to impede public policy aimed at expanding research to find the cause and cure for AD as compared with the assumption of the process as one of culmination of intellectual maturity.

Even when the mind becomes impaired in later life, perspectives and values vary or even confound defining which policy represents the right course of action. Views on the use of life-sustaining interventions for those at an advanced age may confound deliberations on the care of cognitively impaired older adults, as the U.S. Congress's Office of Technology Assessment pointed out in its first comprehensive report on this disease:

> Policy goals presuppose a set of accepted premises. One such premise is that individuals with dementia should be accorded the same respect for their person that they could have expected if they had not lost mental abilities. This does not imply, however, that the same decisions will always be reached—decisions to forgo life-sustaining treatment, for example, may be more acceptable in the presence of irreversible dementia than without it. (Office of Technology Assessment, 1987, p. 4)

VALUES INFLUENCING POLICY

Too often examinations of policy determinations focus only on the debate between *cost* and *quality* of programs being considered. The profound influence of *values*—at times subliminal—is greatly underappreciated.

LESSONS FROM THE PAST

The twenty-five-century-old myth of Tithonus captures the essence of one of the main concerns in the last twenty-five years of the twentieth century. Tithonus, a mere mortal, and Eos, the goddess of dawn, fell hopelessly in love. Eos, desiring to live forever with her lover, pleads with almighty Zeus to bestow the immortality of the gods upon Tithonus. Zeus acquiesced, but in his classic style granted immortality without including eternal youth. Hence, Tithonus proceeded to grow older and older and more and more frail, without dying. The ancient Greeks foresaw the modern person's human dilemma—that progress in extending longevity not outpace progress in improving the quality of added years on later life. Technology's affirmation of whether to enable a longer life has resulted in a struggle to come to terms with how to do so meaningfully.

Some argue that the dilemma of accommodating disability, although a burden for the individual, family, and society, is a historically new phenomenon—that our evolutionary ancestors were pragmatic in the "benign neglect" of disabled elders. But new findings about the Neanderthal society of 100,000 years ago challenge such views, and the fact that these findings come from research on Neanderthals, typically characterized as brutish, makes them even more noteworthy. We now know that the Neanderthals were the first people to regularly bury their dead, regularly take care of their sick and aged. Most skeletons of older Neanderthals show signs of severe impairment, such as withered arms, healed but incapacitated broken bones, tooth loss, and severe osteoarthritis; only care by young Neanderthals could have enabled such older folks to stay alive to the point of such incapacitation (Diamond, 1989, p. 55).

ASPECTS OF ALZHEIMER'S DISEASE INFLUENCING POLICY DEVELOPMENT

A range of phenomena and characteristics of AD influence policies focused on it. Four aspects, in particular, should affect deliberations on research, practice, service development, service delivery, and long-term care.

DISEASE OF UNKNOWN CAUSE

That AD is a disease of unknown cause means that a broad-based research initiative is required—one that follows multiple paths of inquiry. The need to plant a thousand different seeds to cultivate new clues as to the cause of and cure for AD has become recognized. Administratively, this has been translated at the federal level into a coordinated research program involving a partnership of more than a dozen agencies and institutes bringing to bear their unique perspectives and scientific resources. A departmental council has been legislatively established to coordinate this effort, share information, and define new areas of research. As of 1990, the members of this Department of Health and Human Services (DHHS) Council on Alzheimer's Disease included:

- The National Institute on Aging (NIA)
- The National Institute of Mental Health (NIMH)
- The National Institute of Neurological Disorders and Stroke (NINDS)
- The National Institute of Allergy and Infectious Diseases (NIAID)

- The National Center for Nursing Research (NCNR)
- The Agency for Health Care Policy and Research (AHCPR)
- The National Center for Health Statistics (NCHS)
- The Administration on Aging (AOA)
- The Health Resources and Services Administration (HRSA)
- The Health Care Financing Administration (HCFA)
- The Department of Veterans Affairs (VA)
- The Office of the Assistant Secretary for Planning and Evaluation (ASPE)
- The Surgeon General
- The Assistant Secretary for Health (the chairman of the council)

EXCESS DISABILITY—MODIFIABLE SYMPTOMS

Considerable defeatism has accompanied the diagnosis of AD. Because neither the cause of nor the cure for AD is known, many assume that nothing can be done, a notion that could not be further from the truth. Many chronic illnesses lack a cure but benefit from clinical interventions that improve care and/or alleviate significant symptoms; AD is no exception. In this vein, an important clinical phenomenon has been recognized in AD—that of *excess disability*. Excess disability refers to states in the course of AD where coexisting problems compound the dysfunction that the patient experiences from cognitive impairment alone. Depression is a common example; it can coexist with dementia, compounding the patient's overall dysfunction. While no treatment can lift the dementia, intervention can lift the depression, allowing the patient to cope better and suffer less at that point. To the extent that some modification of the patient's symptoms results, family burden may be reduced and the need for nursing home placement postponed. A case example illustrates this clinical phenomenon.

Case Example. A 75-year-old brilliant chemist, Professor Janof, was evaluated because of significant trouble he was having with memory and concentration—to the extent that he no longer could balance his checkbook and no longer took an interest in reading. Professor Janof described difficulty noticeable only to him, a year earlier, when he was becoming less facile with complicated equations. To others he still looked quite sharp, but not to himself. This problem was a terrible blow to his self-esteem, and he began to experience trouble sleeping, loss of appetite and weight, and further difficulty concentrating. A thorough differential diagnostic work-up ruled out many causes of dementia-like symptoms that can mimic senile dementia, and left the clinician with the diagnosis of AD. But the impression was that depression was also present. Treatment was initiated for the depression, combining individual psychotherapy and an antidepressant medication. Professor Janof's appetite returned, the weight loss stopped, concentration improved, he started reading again, though trouble with the checkbook continued. The therapeutic work helped Professor Janof come to terms with his underlying disorder, with AD. Residual skills were maximized during that stage in the course of his disorder; quality of life during that interval was enhanced.

Without an understanding of the potential for excess disability in the course of his disorder, Professor Janof may have been denied a treatment opportunity in the face of a diagnosis of AD. Following the intervention for his depression, another three years passed before he returned to the level of cognitive impairment with which he was first seen clinically. Treatment gave him three better years at a critical juncture in his life course. (Cohen, 1989, p. 153)

In this case example, not only were symptoms modified, but clinical improvement occurred as well, despite an underlying progressive disease process. Moreover, this is not an isolated case example; a series of studies has revealed that the prevalence of excess disability in AD and its response to treatment are much greater than generally realized; indeed, the majority of AD patients have one or more excess-disability–causing problems (Reifler and Larson, 1988; Merriam et al., 1988). More than 30 percent have depression alone, with 85 percent of these individuals responding to therapeutic interventions (Reifler et al., 1986).

The recognition of excess-disability states in AD and their response to clinical interventions have increased the awareness of both the opportunity and the responsibility to treat these patients. Clinical practice and public policy alike are influenced in the process.

A PROGRESSIVE DISORDER WITH A CHANGING CLINICAL PICTURE

Because AD is a progressive disorder with a changing clinical picture, a different range and mix of services at different points during the natural history of the disorder are needed. Symptoms change, the family burden varies, and service settings differ with the progression of AD. Service settings, for example, range from the home, to the community, to the institution. As a result, public policy deliberations at the local, state, and federal levels must all be responsive to the need for a comprehensive set of services and the ability to coordinate them in varying ways depending on individual circumstances.

FAMILY STRESS: THE SECOND PATIENT

Results from studies of family stress in AD reveal that as many as 80 percent of spousal caregivers develop clinically significant symptoms of depression in caring for loved ones with AD (Gallagher, 1987). Moreover, disturbing research findings indicate impaired immune function among family caregivers under chronic stress in providing care for close relatives with AD (Kiecolt-Glaser et al., 1987). The spouse, in effect, often represents the second patient in AD, creating an added public health problem of alarming magnitude. Hence, public policy needs to take into consideration the family system as a whole in AD, with particular attention to the needs of special populations such as ethnic minorities (Valle, 1981; Office of Technology Assessment, 1990).

KEY POLICY DEVELOPMENTS RELATING TO ALZHEIMER'S DISEASE

Key public policy developments relating to AD range from the areas of funding research to financing long-term care.

DIRECTIONS OF RESEARCH: BASIC VERSUS APPLIED

The direction research should follow was one of the early policy debates on AD; should the emphasis be on basic or on applied research? In 1983 then-Secretary of DHHS, Margaret Heckler, established the Secretary's Task Force on Alzheimer's Disease (later legislated into the DHHS Council on Alzheimer's Disease), with the specific goals of coordinating research and defining new research directions. It was quickly recognized that there was no "either/or" resolution in the basic versus applied debate. By definition, basic research is future oriented—it does not bear fruit immediately. Yet appreciation of its role in understanding the causes, cures, and preventions of AD is sometimes lost in the frustration of its lack of applicability to the present—the patients and families burdened with AD today. Clearly, both must be addressed; applied research is required as well to meet the needs of the disease's estimated 4 million victims.

The Secretary's Task Force responded to these concerns by outlining a seven-point research plan, one that still broadly guides present studies (U.S. Department of Health and Human Services, 1984):

- Epidemiology

- Etiology and Pathogenesis

- Diagnosis

- Clinical Course

- Treatment (Pharmacological to Behavioral)

- The Family

- Systems of Care

In the first years following the publication of that report, research mounted in all seven of these domains, but a much greater emphasis was placed on basic research. Congressional concern about adequate emphasis on applied studies—especially services research—led to the Alzheimer's Disease and Related Dementias Services Research Act of 1986 (Title IX of Public Law 99-660). P.L. 99-660 mandated services research within four agencies of the Department of Health and Human Services: the National Institute on Aging, the National Institute of Mental Health, the Agency for Health Care Policy and Research (called the National Center for Health Services Research and Health Care Technology Assessment at the time of the legislation), and the Health Care Financing Administration.

MAGNITUDE OF RESEARCH SUPPORT

In 1976 less than $4 million per year went to federally supported research on AD. By 1989 that figure had reached $130 million. But the rate of increase then leveled off, despite the concurrent explosion of new findings and scientific talent in AD studies. This discrepancy, in part explained by national budgetary problems, came under the scrutiny of the congressionally appointed Advisory Panel on Alzheimer's Disease, established by the same legislation named above. The advisory panel was charged with making policy recommendations in the areas of biomedical research, services research, the provision of services, and the financing of services for Alzheimer victims and their families. The panel highlighted the need for more research support, expressed concern about the flattening of the funding curve, and recommended $350 million per year for AD research at the start of the 1990s (U.S. Department of Health and Human Services, 1989). Moreover, the advisory panel suggested that the level of federal support for research on Alzheimer's should be comparable in magnitude to levels provided for other diseases of major public health concern.

Interestingly, the panel's research-support recommendations are conservative in relation to those put forth in legislative bills by various members of Congress. Moreover, the Pepper Commission (the U.S. Bipartisan Commission on Comprehensive Health Care, charged with making recommendations to Congress on "access to health care and long-term care for all Americans") recommended a research agenda on long-term care with an annual funding of $1 billion; the areas emphasized for study were predominantly those of AD and related problems of older adults.

LONG-TERM CARE INSURANCE

AD, more than any other disorder, is pushing the need for long-term care insurance, since between half and two-thirds of those in nursing homes have AD or a related dementia.

Wrong-Term Care Insurance. A growing policy issue and values concern is that the most affluent country in the world does not have an adequate and affordable long-term care insurance for its general population. Important to note is that most Americans are not aware of this, the vast majority incorrectly thinking that Medicare provides such coverage (Williams and Katzman, 1988). Unfortunately, when it comes to chronic illness, most older Americans have "wrong-term" care insurance. Meanwhile, intense study is under way to rectify this situation, with careful scrutiny of which long-term care services might be covered and what mechanisms might be used to finance them (Capitman, 1990).

S-ADLs. Part of current policy deliberations on who would qualify for long-term care insurance benefits has focused on eligibility criteria using the standard of specific number of impaired activities of daily living (ADLs); ADLs are basic tasks of everyday life such as dressing, bathing, and eating. But ADL scales alone do not provide sufficient criteria for determining long-term care service eligibility, and their use poses a distinct problem for Alzheimer's disease and related dementia patients. While many such patients are physically able to perform ADLs, supervision and cueing (prompting by others) are often necessary to ensure that they actually accomplish such daily living activities and to ensure their safety and that of others around them. Therefore, eligibility criteria based on ADLs need to be supplemented with provisions that recognize the special dependencies created by patients with need for cueing and supervision (see U.S. Department of Health and Human Services, 1989).

Perhaps one could consider S-ADLs (supervised-ADLs) in establishing eligibility criteria—that is, ADLs that would be compromised in the absence of supervision, to the extent that the patient could not adequately carry them out.

SERVICES IN THE COMMUNITY VERSUS SERVICES IN INSTITUTIONS

Apart from cost versus appropriate care views, there is the matter of values that influence decisions about living arrangements—about whether AD patients should reside in the community or in a nursing home. It is important to recognize, however, that there are growing AD populations in both community and institutional settings—approximately a million in nursing homes, but nearly three times that number in the community. Hence, any balanced program would need to address both groups. Policymakers have only recently become aware of the vast numbers of families burdened with AD in the community and the strong desire of family members to keep those with the disorder at home as long as possible. The Omnibus Budget Reconciliation Act of 1986 addresses the strong orientation toward helping AD patients to remain in the community by mandating a three-year, $40-million Medicare Alzheimer's Disease Demonstration of community-based comprehensive services, as does a major $4.2-million Robert Wood Johnson Foundation demonstration project (Office of Technology Assessment, 1990).

TRAINING

Training for both researchers and practitioners is receiving increasing attention in policy deliberations (U.S. Department of Health and Human Services, 1989). The Advisory Panel on Alzheimer's Disease, for example, has emphasized the need in future directions of research to enlarge the pool of new investigators trained in state-of-the-art molecular biology, quantitative pathology, and clinical investigative techniques. In addition, the panel has stressed the importance of clinical training not only for the range of health care professionals who treat AD patients, but for family caregivers as well. As activity mounts in the area of clinical personnel, concerns about credentialing and licensing will add to the challenge of developing the best overall plan for preparing providers of care.

CONCLUSION

There's an old admonition that asserts that "for every complicated problem there's a simple solution . . . and, that simple solution always fails." The varied natural history of AD, its changing clinical picture with a different range and mix of needed services during its progression, the location of large numbers of AD patients in both community and nursing home settings, and the fact that patient and family alike demand major attention by service providers force the realization that AD is not a simple problem, and current policy deliberations must reflect an awareness of its complexity.

REFERENCES

Capitman, J.A. (1990). Policy and program options in community-oriented long-term care. In M.P. Lawton, ed., *Annual Review of Gerontology and Geriatrics*, Vol. 9, pp. 357–388. New York: Springer Publishing Co.

Cohen, G.D. (1989). *The Brain in Human Aging*. New York: Springer Publishing Co.

Diamond, J. (1989). The great leap forward. *Discover, 10:*50–60.

Gallagher, D. (1987). Caregivers of chronically ill elders. In G.L. Maddox, ed., *The Encyclopedia of Aging*, pp. 89–91. New York: Springer Publishing Co.

Kane, R.A. (1986). Senile dementia and public policy. In M.L.M. Gilhooly, S.H. Zarit, and J.E. Birren, eds., *The Dementias: Policy and Management*, pp. 190–214. Englewood Cliffs, N.J.: Prentice-Hall.

Kiecolt-Glaser, J.K., Glaser, R., Dyer, C., Shuttleworth, E.C., Ogrocki, P., and Speicher, C.E. (1987). Chronic stress and immune function in family caregivers of Alzheimer disease victims. *Psychosomatic Medicine, 49:*523–535.

Merriam, A.E., Aronson, M.K., Gaston, P., Wey, S., and Katz, I. (1988). The psychiatric symptoms of Alzheimer's disease. *Journal of the American Geriatrics Society, 36:*7–12.

Office of Technology Assessment, Congress of the United States. (1987). *Losing a Million Minds: Confronting the Tragedy of Alzheimer's Disease and Other Dementias*. Washington, D.C.: U.S. Government Printing Office.

Office of Technology Assessment, Congress of the United States. (1990). *Confused Minds, Burdened Families: Finding Help for People with Alzheimer's Disease*. Washington, D.C.: U.S. Government Printing Office.

Reifler, B.V., and Larson, E. (1988). Excess disability in demented elderly outpatients: the rule of the halves. *Journal of the American Geriatrics Society, 36:*82–83.

Reifler, B.V., Larson, E., Teri, L., and Poulsen, M. (1986). Dementia of the Alzheimer's type and depression. *Journal of the American Geriatrics Society, 34:*855–859.

U.S. Department of Health and Human Services. (1984). *Report of the Secretary's Task Force on Alzheimer's Disease* (DHHS Publication No. ADM 84-1323). Washington, D.C.: U.S. Government Printing Office.

U.S. Department of Health and Human Services. (1989). *Report of the Advisory Panel on Alzheimer's Disease* (DHHS Publication No. ADM 89-1644). Washington, D.C.: U.S. Government Printing Office.

Valle, R. (1981). Natural support systems, minority groups, and the late life dementias: implications for service delivery, research, and policy. In G.D. Cohen and N.E. Miller, eds., *Clinical Aspects of Alzheimer's Disease and Senile Dementia*, pp. 277–299. New York: Raven Press.

Williams, T.F., and Katzman, B. (1988). Public policy issues. In L.F. Jarvik and C.H. Winograd, eds., *Treatment for the Alzheimer Patient*, pp. 147–154. New York: Springer Publishing Co.

INDEX

AARP. *See* American Association for Retired Persons
Acetylcholine, 27
Adkins, Janet, 101–3
Advance directives, 12–13, 74, 91–92, 93–94, 95
Alzheimer, Alois, 23
Alzheimer's Association, 5, 6
Alzheimer's disease: biological features of, 25–26; changing needs of people with, 175–76; diagnosis of, 23, 27, 32; euthanasia in advanced cases of, 118–37; experience of, 31–36; genetic forms of, 25–26; impact of, on family, 176; increased awareness of, 5; nature of, 11; prevalence of, 146; and public policy, 171–79; research issues related to, 26–28, 173–74, 177–78, 179; resource allocation for people with, 124–27; symptoms of, 23–25, 174–75; and training for caregivers, 179. *See also* Dementia
Alzheimer's Disease and Related Dementias Services Research Act of 1986, 177
American Association for Retired Persons (AARP), 6, 164
American Medical Association, guidelines on treatment, 103
Amnesia, as symptom of dementia, 24

Arras, John, 76–77
Autonomy: bioethical perspective on, 90–92; as issue in active euthanasia, 119–22; as issue in treatment decision-making, 73–75, 83–84, 86–87; and right to die, 104

Balk, Alfred, 157
Barber v. Superior Court, 75
Battin, Margaret P., 13, 64, 103
Behavior, as indicative of dementia, 44–45. *See also* Personality
Beneficence, as issue in euthanasia, 88–90, 94
Bernlef, J., 38
Binstock, Robert H., 14–15
Bioethics, 86–87; problems with dominant model of, 88–93. *See also* Communicative ethics; Moral issues
Bipartisan Commission on Comprehensive Health Care (Pepper Commission), 10, 149
Boffey, Phillip, 49
Bopp, James, 111, 113
Bowen, Otis, 163
British National Health Service, 158
Brody, Elaine M., 61–62
Bronte, D. Lydia, 63
Buchanan, Allen, 74
Buchanan, James, 86

Designed by Christopher Harris/Summer Hill Books
Composed by Achorn Graphics in Janson text
and Helvetica Thin display.
Printed on 60 lb. Glatfelter Offset, A-50
by The Maple Press Company.